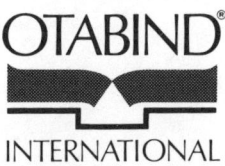
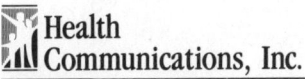
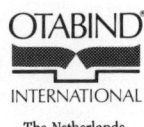

ROMANCE TO DIE FOR

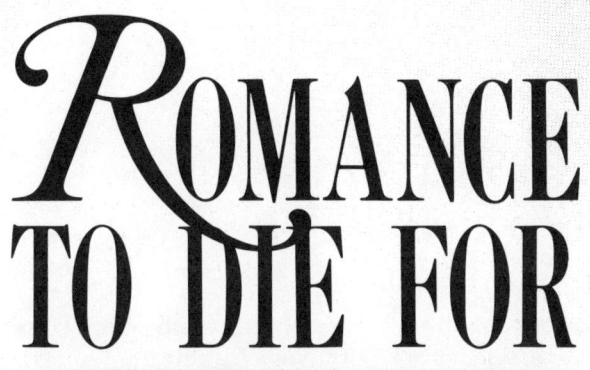

ROMANCE TO DIE FOR

The Startling Truth About Women, Sex And AIDS

FLEUR SACK, M.D.

with Anne Streeter

Health Communications, Inc.
Deerfield Beach, Florida

Library of Congress Cataloging-in-Publication Data

Sack, Fleur, 1948—
    Romance to die for: the startling truth about women, sex,
and AIDS/Fleur Sack with Anne Streeter.
      p.   cm.
    Includes bibliographical references.
    ISBN 1-55874-240-9
    1. AIDS (Disease) — Popular works. 2. Safe sex in AIDS
prevention. 3. Women — Diseases. I. Streeter, Anne.
1951 — II. Title.
RC607.A26S22   1992   92-32159
616.97′92′0082—dc20   CIP

©1992 Fleur Sack with Anne Streeter
ISBN 1-55874-240-9

Publisher: Health Communications, Inc.
              3201 S.W. 15th Street
              Deerfield Beach, Florida 33442-8190

Cover design by Barbara Bergman

DEDICATION

This book is dedicated to all the compassionate health-care workers, social workers and volunteers who care for AIDS patients, giving of themselves until there is no more to give; and to the all too many individuals who have lived with the horror of HIV disease.

$\mathcal{A}$CKNOWLEDGMENTS

Even in this busy world, if something is important enough, people make time to do whatever is necessary to help out.

That's been especially true in writing this book. Many people — all busy professionals — made time to make sure the information presented in this book is both timely and informative. I am very grateful for their contributions.

Anne Streeter was as committed as I was to the writing of this book. As Administrative Director of Women's Services at Baptist Hospital of Miami and a former health care journalist, she was well-prepared to help me with the presenting and polishing of the manuscript. I would like to thank her for the tireless energy she devoted to this book, and to thank her husband, Bill Streeter, for his support.

I wish to acknowledge Barbara Nichols, my editor at Health Communications, who was truly committed to seeing this book published, and who provided valuable insight into what women today would want to know about HIV disease and AIDS. Thanks also to Peter Vegso, Health Communications' publisher, who is using the power of the press to save lives.

Special thanks are also due to the many women who have shared their stories with me, and to the healthcare professionals who offered their assistance, including Patti Wetzel, a physician infected with HIV; Ellen Bukstel-Segal, a widow whose husband died from AIDS; Barbara Russell, an infection control nurse at Baptist Hospital; psychologist Suzanne Keeley; Diane Ream and her staff in the Health Science Library at Baptist Hospital of Miami; Catherine G. Lynch of the Miami Health Crisis Network and Bruce Lenes, M.D., of the South Florida Red Cross.

I would also like to thank my colleague and friend, Dr. Allan Stein, who shared his knowledge, emotions and office with me while this epidemic unfolded in our practices. My staff need to be acknowledged for being true heroines. Taking care of dying patients is never easy but they have done that with compassion and dedication. I am especially grateful for the enthusiastic support they gave me during the writing of this book.

I want to thank my husband, Simon, my sons, Terry and Gary Frank, and my mother, Ray Sack, not only for their advice and patience during the days and nights spent writing this book, but also for their understanding of my commitment to this epidemic.

CONTENTS

Introduction xi

1. Romance To Die For 1
2. AIDS: What It Is And How It Started 15
3. Getting Attention For Women 29
4. From Person To Person 41
5. Deadly Betrayals 49
6. Why People Take Risks 59
7. Romance To Live For 75
8. Testing: The Only Way You'll
   Know For Sure (Maybe!) 87
9. Use Your Condom Sense 103
10. And Baby Makes Three 123
11. Teens: Our Future At Risk 135
12. Other Sexually Transmitted Diseases 147
13. Safety Of The Healthcare Setting:
    Two Sides Of The Coin 165
14. Blood: A Life-Sustaining Force 177
15. Myths, Questions And Answers About AIDS ... 191
16. What Can You Do? Spread Information,
    Not AIDS 201

Appendix 1: Glossary 211

          2: HIV/AIDS Resource Directory 219

Bibliography 221

$\mathcal{I}$NTRODUCTION

In 1985 I treated my first AIDS patient and the experience changed my life.

By the time I met Gary, a bright and talented musician, at the hospital where I work, there was nothing I could do to help him except to make his hospital stay as comfortable as possible in his last weeks of life.

I spent hours talking with this kind 26-year-old man, getting to know about his life and how this disease had affected him. After the second day, I realized that Gary had no visitors, which seemed odd. He was a friendly, open young man, the sort of fellow who is usually surrounded by friends.

"Gary, don't you have any friends in this city?" I asked.

"Dr. Sack," he said simply, "all my friends are dead."

I was stunned. Suddenly, the full implications of the medical journal reports I had been reading — as if they were distant abstractions — hit home. This was a vicious disease that was spreading faster than anyone could have predicted, leaving in its wake the anguish of pain and suffering, hopelessness and despair.

I soon began to observe that while most people read about AIDS in the press and see occasional reports on television, the terrible horror of the situation remains undigested. It doesn't register that AIDS can happen to anyone. To them.

My teenage son is a perfect example. For years he had heard me talk about AIDS, but when Magic Johnson spoke out about his condition, my son was surprised.

"Gee, Mom," he said, "I guess heterosexuals *can* get AIDS."

I was floored. My husband is also a doctor, and we thought we had made the dangers of AIDS perfectly clear to our children. All I could think was, *What on earth will it take to wake people up?*

Immunity To Information

Every day in my medical practice I see evidence that people tend to develop an immunity to information they don't want to think about. Patients who should know better and protect themselves test positive for HIV, the virus that causes AIDS. Surprisingly, many of these patients are well-educated mainstream women. Their minds may deny the threat of AIDS, but the virus won't be denied by their bodies. HIV has respect for neither status nor education level.

Part of the confusion stems from the early years of the AIDS epidemic when it seemed to be a disease that for the most part infected gay men. But increasingly we are seeing women who have been infected — often by the men they love.

Since treating Gary in 1985, I've seen many aspects of AIDS and the people who get it. In the hospital I've held the hands of dying patients and cried with their heartbroken families and friends. In my family practice I've seen teenage girls who don't understand anything about AIDS even though they have had some AIDS education in school. I've seen mothers who worry about their children but do not protect themselves. And I've seen the "worried well," women who are terrified that they, their family or friends may be infected.

I know how confused and afraid women are.

We have good reason to be. The latest study on world-wide AIDS conducted by the Harvard School of Public Health produced some terrifying statistics. By the year 2000 as many as 110 million people may be infected with the AIDS virus. At least 40 percent of them will be women. This disease is rapidly becoming the most threatening killer the world has ever known, far worse than the Bubonic Plague, which decimated the population of Europe in the 14th century.

The shocking truth is that there are no real experts on AIDS in women because until recently drug research projects failed to reach or serve women. We are just beginning to learn it is easier for women to contract AIDS through sexual intercourse than it is for men and are just now discovering the effect of AIDS medications on women.

The only weapon we have against AIDS is information. We can't cure the disease yet, but we can *prevent* it.

For years I have been lecturing to doctors and educators and continue to speak before various groups of adults and children. I've lectured in South Africa, my native country and where I was educated, and have been featured on Good Morning, South Africa. I've even had meetings with tribal witch doctors in Zululand to try to impress upon them the importance of AIDS prevention — an exercise as futile as trying to convince the Reagan and Bush administrations to provide funding for AIDS research.

Sometimes I feel I am fighting a losing battle. In my family practice and in my hospital, I see more and more people test positive for HIV and greater numbers dying of AIDS every day.

I hope the information in this book will help you to understand AIDS and to avoid it at any cost. You don't have to die of AIDS. Now that we understand how the virus is transmitted, in almost all instances you have to

be a willing participant to acquire this disease. The choice
is yours.

Please, love carefully.

Fleur Sack, M.D.
Miami, Florida

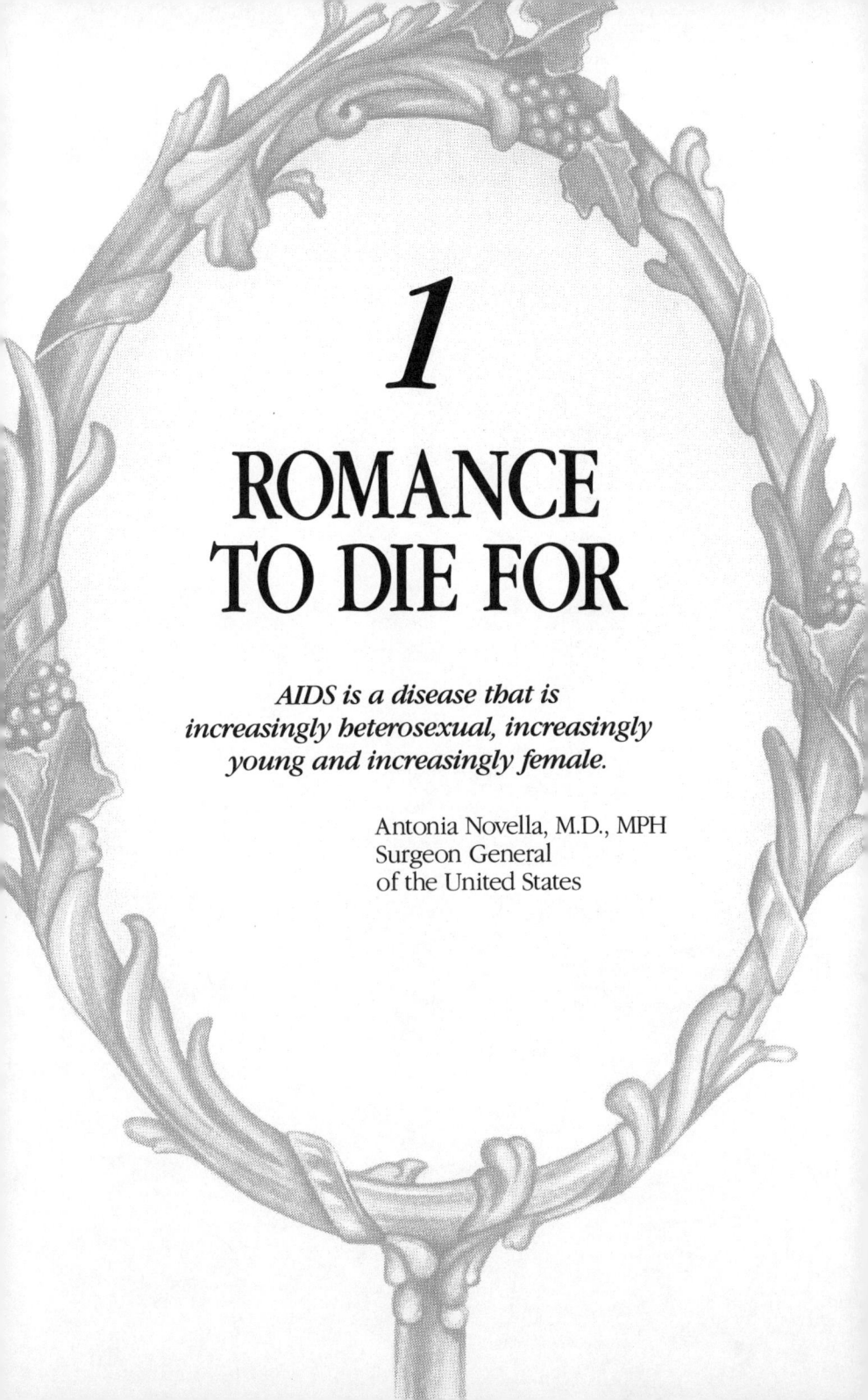

1
ROMANCE
TO DIE FOR

*AIDS is a disease that is
increasingly heterosexual, increasingly
young and increasingly female.*

Antonia Novella, M.D., MPH
Surgeon General
of the United States

*I*n thousands of bookstores around the world you can find shelf after shelf filled with romance novels, their covers adorned with impossibly beautiful women and incredibly handsome men in a lavish setting. Romance novels have always sold well, fueling the fantasies and satisfying the emotional needs of their readers. Romance is so glamorous, so exciting.

A common thread runs through many of these stories: They meet. She distrusts him. He forces her to have sex with him against her wishes. She hates it at the beginning, but finds herself melting into him and becomes his woman right then and there. They go off to have adventures which usually include her taming him into a kind, considerate, responsible, yet passionate husband.

These "bodice-rippers" are obviously works of fiction. But many women, whether or not they read romance novels, truly believe in the romance myth — or at least hope it's true. Love will win out over everything. If I'm a wonderful girlfriend or wife, it will all turn out fine in the end.

Today these beliefs may be dangerous. Consider the case of socialite Mary Fisher, whose real life is more glamorous than most romance writers could imagine. The radiantly beautiful daughter of a philanthropic family travels in prominent circles, insulated by everything the world has to offer — money, power, position. In February 1992 *The Miami Herald* reported that Ms. Fisher had the Human Immunodeficiency Virus (HIV). It seems that when she divorced her husband after a three-year marriage, he left her the house, their two young sons — and the AIDS virus. He didn't know until after their divorce that he had been infected with the virus. At his urging, she was tested and discovered that she was infected too.

She told the interviewer, "I wasn't gay. I didn't use drugs. I wasn't a prostitute . . . I would think of it from time to time and then dismiss it by taking myself out of those categories."

Now she knows better. "It can happen to anyone," she said. "I was infected in a loving, trusting relationship."

Mary Fisher is a brave, compassionate woman. She didn't need to make her tragedy known to the public, but we should be grateful that she did, for her story will help save lives.

Since I began caring for people with HIV disease, I have seen growing numbers of educated, vivacious, well-to-do women become infected with the virus that kills. Some were married, some divorced, some were involved with multiple partners. All of their stories are startling, but I doubt that the press would cover them. To get attention in the media, it seems, you have to be star material. I wonder all the time at the mind-set of people running television networks.

If an enormous asteroid from deep space was on a collision course with Planet Earth and was certain to kill millions of people when it struck, the media coverage would be constant with news updates every day. Indeed, the AIDS virus is just as dramatic and serious a crisis, yet it doesn't rate a high priority for coverage. Why?

Let's take a look at the priorities of the networks. The day the Harvard School of Public Health announced its new projections on the spread of AIDS, the new Elvis Presley stamp was also announced. A friend of mine who was home with the flu that day was flipping through the TV channels for something interesting to watch and said she saw a report of the AIDS figures only once, while the Elvis Presley postage stamp was discussed hour after hour all around the dial.

If you don't think AIDS is a crisis, consider the Harvard numbers. By 2000, as many as 110 million people in the world will be infected with the HIV virus. More than 40 percent, or about 44 million of them, are likely to be women. Eventually, all of them will suffer and die.

While there are many aspects of this disease the medical profession does not know, we do know that AIDS is rapidly becoming a disease of women. When this epidemic first started in the early 1980s, only two percent of those infected in the United States were women. As of March 1992, 12 percent of those infected were women. In Puerto Rico the number is 18 percent.

Worldwide the infection rate among women is expected to pass the rate for men by the year 2000. At the 8th International Conference on AIDS in July 1992, 20 sessions were devoted to women, an enormous change from previous conferences when women were almost ignored. It is clear that women need to take the AIDS problem very seriously.

Nice Girls Do

Probably more than half the women diagnosed with sexually transmitted AIDS got it from their husbands or from men they have lived with for years. Many of these women are not the IV drug users who are so prone to being infected with the AIDS virus through sharing dirty needles. Rather, they are women whose husbands or lovers were infected and perhaps unknowingly transmitted the virus through unprotected sex.

The last three new women patients I've seen with AIDS were all married to loving partners: one to a former IV drug user with years in recovery; one to a man who had a contaminated blood transfusion in 1985; and one to a man who had been divorced and had other sex partners prior to their marriage. These women believed in love and romance and felt safe and protected by their marriages from any outside threat.

What they didn't bargain on was a tiny virus that doesn't care about the love two people have for each other. This virus is concerned only about finding a way into another body and destroying the body's magnificent means of fighting disease.

As long as the myth prevails that women who are in committed relationships with men are safe from AIDS, we will be unable to stop the epidemic from spreading. And women will continue to be infected faster than men.

In the United States AIDS is already the fifth leading cause of death in women ages 15 to 44 — women who are in the prime of their childbearing years. HIV-infected women who become pregnant have about a 30 percent chance of passing this disease on to their babies.

If you think that love and romance will protect you from AIDS, think again. It's estimated that 1.5 million people in America were infected with HIV by 1992. One out of every 800 women and one out of every 100 men has HIV disease. Unfortunately, not all of those people know they are infected and may be unwittingly spreading this killer disease to those they love through sexual intercourse or the sharing of needles used for drug injection. People with HIV disease will go on to develop AIDS and virtually all will die from infections that will ravage their bodies.

I know that statistics can be numbing so I want to give you some case histories of women who are, or have been, my patients.

The Wedding Bells Toll For Thee

Sherry was a beautiful 25-year-old woman with loving parents, a handsome husband and a great future planned. Sherry and Stan had been married for a year when she started talking about wanting a family.

Stan avoided conversations about having a baby and discussing it became increasingly difficult. Sherry kept bringing up the subject until one day he told her the reason for his reluctance.

Eight years before, as a young college student, he had tried using IV drugs. It went on for just a short time before his family realized what was going on and got him into recovery. He'd been completely rehabilitated for years and vowed to put it all behind him. He would never discuss this awful period in his life with anyone, not even Sherry. But recent media attention on AIDS was haunting him. He felt and looked perfectly well but because of his drug abuse history, he felt he should be tested for HIV before they had children.

I'll never forget the day this beautiful young couple came into my office for the results of their tests and I had to tell them they both tested HIV positive. They were devastated, and so was I.

Watching Sherry die was one of the most anguishing experiences of my life. After her diagnosis, she deteriorated very rapidly into full-blown AIDS. She became an emaciated 85-pound wraith who suffered severe bouts of diarrhea up to 24 times a day. She had sores in her mouth, constant pain, high fevers and various infections.

Stan and Sherry moved in with her parents because she needed almost full-time care for months before she died. It took all three of them plus occasional nursing care and intermittent hospitalization to get her through the last months of her life. It was doubly difficult watching Sherry's parents as they took care of her. They were lovely people and, like most of us affected by this epidemic, did not deserve the heartbreak that had been thrust upon them.

The last time I saw Stan, he was still healthy and handsome. Even though the HIV virus had been in his system years longer than it had been in Sherry's, he remained well. He has moved out of his in-laws' house because it was awkward to bring new girlfriends into their home. I told him he must, by law, tell his prospective lovers of his HIV status and advised him to use condoms if they chose to go to bed with him. I can only hope that he is taking my advice. And if I could speak with his new girlfriends, I would advise them not to get sexually involved with him at all. I'd prefer that no one have sex with a known carrier of this dread disease.

It's impossible to know why Sherry's husband remained healthy while she died. However, it's not an unusual case. Often, the partners of IV drug abusers get sicker sooner than the abuser himself. But there is no doubt that he, too, will eventually die of this disease.

Unfortunately Sherry is just one of the thousands of women in this country and of millions in the world who have unknowingly been condemned to a horrible death through an act of love.

Getting Involved With Mr. Wrong

One of my patients at high risk for getting HIV was married to a bisexual man and is now having an affair with a married man. Her story is both fascinating and frustrating to me.

Susan is a 45-year-old professional woman, with a master's degree and a very active, full life. After 21 years of marriage, her husband confessed to her that he was bisexual and had had a male lover for some time. He decided that he was not willing to give up his male partner. Susan felt she had no option but to divorce him, though she cared for him deeply. She took an HIV test and fortunately tested negative.

Several months after her divorce, Susan was involved in a car accident. Tom, a paramedic, came to help her and escorted her home as she was very shaken. He called on her and visited her several times after that. Their friendship soon turned into a romance. She had previously had only one sex partner, her husband, and although having an affair with a married man was not her style, she was lonely, vulnerable and in love. Tom told her he had never had an affair and had a satisfactory marriage.

I met Susan when she came for testing, feeling angry, betrayed and scared. After two years of romancing her, Tom confessed that he was HIV infected. He said he had acquired the virus from an infected accident victim whom he had assisted several years previously. He hadn't told her about this before because he was afraid it would interfere with their love affair and that he would lose her.

Tom had, however, shared this information with his wife, and they were no longer having sex.

It was an emotional interview for me. I empathized with Susan's feelings of terror. And I was surprised at the depth of the anger I felt toward Tom. I felt he should be convicted for attempted manslaughter.

Again Susan tested negative. But that's not the end of the story. Susan has returned to see me three times since for testing. She is still having sex with Tom, still in love with him and he is now living with her. His wife learned of the affair and demanded that Tom leave the house. And my patient is now his caregiver, his lover and his friend.

Susan is still testing negative for HIV, but chances are that she won't remain uninfected. If she does acquire the virus, by the time she gets AIDS, Tom will be long dead, and I wonder who will be Susan's caregiver, lover and friend.

I wonder if Susan really believes this is a romance worth dying for. I imagine at some level of her consciousness she feels completely overwhelmed, believing she just can't escape the virus. First her husband, then her lover have put her life in jeopardy. It's a lot like the Country and Western song, "Love Hurts," another romantic myth similar to the plot lines of bodice-ripper novels. But love doesn't have to hurt, believe me. If Susan were thinking clearly, I believe she would stop the affair or at least stop having sex with him.

A woman who has a hard time saying no to a dangerous situation probably ought to have psychological counseling. She might also attend meetings of Co-dependents Anonymous, a 12-Step support group for people who are self-sacrificing to the point of self-destruction. It's possible she would find the strength to leave this man who so dangerously betrayed her. At this point she is not psychologically strong enough to act in her own best interests.

Incomprehensible Promiscuity

Many people, including a doctor friend, look dumbfounded when I tell them people who are HIV positive still go out and play the field. "Surely they stop when they find out they're infected," they usually exclaim. It's a dangerous assumption.

Penny is a 42-year-old mother of a 21-year-old daughter. After her divorce from Dave, Penny had a number of sex partners. Two years later, she found out that she was HIV infected. Thinking back carefully, Penny believes one of her lovers may have been gay. But she doesn't know how to contact him now.

Penny cried for half an hour on the telephone when making her first appointment to see me. She had just received the results of her test and was overwhelmed by the news. My secretary was almost in tears when she told me about my new patient.

Penny sobbed for the first hour of our appointment and couldn't hear anything I had to say. We made another appointment two days later. This was more than a year ago. Penny has since learned a lot about living with the virus. She's HIV infected but relatively healthy at present. She has a full-time job and volunteers to talk to school kids about this disease. She has been reconciled with her ex-husband, who is loving and supportive. Dave has been tested for the virus and has learned all about safer sex practices. He decided to continue to have a sexual relationship with Penny.

At her last office visit, Penny told me she now has two other lovers. She has told most of her friends that she is HIV infected and some, she says, "Have dropped me like a ton of bricks." But these two men in her life know that she's HIV infected and still choose to have sex with her. She says they always wear condoms.

At present, life feels rich and rewarding to Penny. I can't help wondering why anyone who knows she is HIV positive would continue to have sex with her at all. But it is, I understand, a complicated issue.

If you are infected, please tell your sexual partners. It is illegal not to.

When She Was Good, She Was Very, Very Good

In some ways I had great admiration for Wendy, a 25-year-old recovering drug addict who earned her living through prostitution. She was very cute and quite charming. Once she found out that she was HIV positive, she tried to turn her life around. She went back to get her high school diploma and devoted the remaining days of her life to lecturing young people about the dangers of IV drug abuse and teaching them about safer sex. She was supported by a man she met and married, even though the marriage was unable to sustain the difficulties of her disease.

Wendy was charming and responsible when she was not using drugs. But her recovery was hard for her to sustain and she was quite different when she relapsed into drug abuse. I know that when she was really high, she forgot to practice safer sex, and though she wouldn't admit it, I wouldn't be surprised if she shared needles. Perhaps she even practiced her old profession again. I can't help but wonder how many people this patient infected. Wendy died alone in her home last week.

Suicidal Sex: The Ultimate Denial

For many women, taking care of those they love is the great joy in their lives. They are wonderful wives and mothers and considerate allies, delightful co-workers, always ready to go out of their way to do a kindness for a friend. Healthy nurturing is one of the great gifts women have. But when caring for others goes to such an extreme that you lose all sense of yourself, it becomes a kind of human sacrifice — quite literally if AIDS is in the picture.

A new AIDS patient came to my office. Harvey is separated from his wife and five children, and brought with him a woman he described to me as "my significant other." I turned to her and said, "Significant Other, are you practicing safe sex?" Apparently, I opened a can of worms because Harvey jumped in and said, "Talk to her, Dr. Sack. Tell her she needs to be careful."

I asked her if they always used a condom. Joan answered, "Most of the time, but I don't really believe that I'll ever become infected."

When I asked her why, Joan sighed deeply and said, "I've gone through so much in my life, I don't think I'll also get AIDS."

I asked her, "Do you think the AIDS virus is going to say, 'Lady, you've gone through so much, I think I'll leave you alone and infect somebody else'?"

Joan looked at me and said, "You don't understand. Harvey is all I've got."

I realized there was no way I could break through Joan's denial of her risk in the next ten minutes — to teach her enough self-esteem to believe that her life was worth protecting; to make her feel that life was worthwhile to her, even without having suicidal sex with Harvey. Talk about romance to die for.

I needed something to get Joan's attention — and, with sudden insight, I found it. "He needs you to take care of him," I said. "You can't afford to get sick."

That got to her. She made an appointment for testing and for education.

The Equal-Opportunity Virus

Any sexually active woman who feels she's not at risk is not facing the facts. This is an equal opportunity virus. It doesn't care what color you are, how old you are or how much money you have in the bank. It's not impressed with how often you go to church, how good, nice, charitable or socially prominent you are. How hard or easy your life has been doesn't mean a thing to HIV. Sadly, even loyal wives are not necessarily protected from it.

As I become more deeply involved with the epidemic, I see that one of the most dangerous facets of the spread of disease is women's feeling of powerlessness. Women's Liberation has made great strides — we have women astronauts and senators and doctors everywhere, but in my experience I see even well-educated professional women still feel powerless when it comes to their romantic relationships with men.

Learning to find the courage to say no and mean it is much more difficult than any "Just Say No" slogan can convey. But in this age of AIDS, "No" may be the most important word in your vocabulary.

If you are a woman who has trouble saying no to your husband or lover, perhaps you should seek help and guidance from a professional counselor or a support group.

2
AIDS:
WHAT IT IS AND
HOW IT STARTED

*Infection with the AIDS virus
is potentially lethal to all women and
children, irrespective of lifestyle
or sexual activity.*

Dr. John Seale,
Venereologist

*B*efore continuing the story of women and AIDS, we need to back up a bit to look at the origins of the disease and make some definitions clear.

First of all, AIDS is an acronym for *Acquired Immune Deficiency Syndrome*. These four words explain exactly what AIDS is:

- *Acquired* refers to the fact that AIDS is something you get from someone else or from blood. You do not inherit AIDS as you, for example, inherit the color of your hair.
- *Immune* means protected. If you are immune to a disease, you are protected from getting it. Your immune system stops germs from multiplying and infecting your body.
- *Deficiency* means lack of or a shortage. A person with AIDS is immune deficient. That is, the person's immune system does not work properly and is not protecting that person from diseases.
- *Syndrome* is a group of symptoms or problems. If you have AIDS you can get swollen

glands, have weight loss, fever, diarrhea and certain unusual infections and cancers that do not infect people whose immune systems are healthy. A person with AIDS can have one disease or cancer or several diseases and cancers at the same time.

HIV stands for *Human Immunodeficiency Virus*. It is the name of the virus that causes AIDS, just as the chicken pox virus causes chicken pox. These three words describe this virus:

- *Human* means people, not animals, plants or insects.
- *Immunodeficiency* means that a person's immune system is damaged and can't fight off diseases well.
- *Virus* is a tiny germ able to cause diseases.

HIV *infected* means that once the virus invades the body — unlike other viruses, such as those causing colds and flu — it does not leave. It stays in the body forever, using the body's own cells to make copies of itself. It keeps on reproducing. Each of the infected cells, in fact, becomes a little HIV factory.

HIV primarily invades *T-helper cells*, which are white blood cells responsible for helping the body fight off disease. These T-helper cells (also called CD-4 cells) are taken over by HIV and keep on multiplying. Ultimately, the T-helper cells are destroyed, and additional viruses are released in the body, attacking new T-helper cells.

HIV can also infect and destroy other cells in the body, such as those in the brain. That is why some people with AIDS lose their memory, have difficulty performing tasks which they could easily cope with previously or have mental disorders.

HIV Antibodies

Whenever you are infected with a virus or bacteria, your body produces antibodies specifically against that particular germ. Usually these antibodies help protect you from getting reinfected or ill from that germ.

From three weeks to six weeks after being infected with HIV, your body will produce antibodies specifically against HIV. However, unlike other antibodies, these will not protect you from becoming ill. They can't stop the virus from invading cells and reproducing. These unique antibodies are, however, useful in helping doctors determine if you have been infected with HIV. Doctors use a simple blood test to check for HIV antibodies. If antibodies are found, the result is called HIV positive, meaning the person is infected and has *seroconverted*. If antibodies are not found, the result is called HIV negative.

The Window Period

Because it takes time for the body to manufacture HIV antibodies, there is a *"window period"* — the time between when you are infected and when enough antibodies are in your body to show up on the blood test. This window period lasts anywhere from three weeks to six months.

For example, assume you had sex on a Friday night with an infected individual, and you became infected with the virus. If you went to be tested for the virus during the next week, the results would be negative. This is because your body would not have had time to produce antibodies. In spite of the HIV negative report (and in spite of the relief you may feel at getting that report), you would actually be infected and could infect others.

However, anywhere from three weeks to six months later, your body will have produced antibodies. When you are retested, you would be found to be HIV positive. If there is any possibility at all that you are infected, it is vital to be tested and then retested if you think you were infected less than six months before your first test.

Do not confuse this with the time it may take before you get sick. It could take months or many years after infection before you become ill, but your test will be positive by six months after infection.

The Stages Of HIV Disease

Once you are infected with HIV, you can go through several stages in what is called the HIV spectrum of diseases. They are:

Initial Stage or Stage 1 — Within three to four weeks of infection, a newly infected person may have a flulike illness with fever, occasionally enlarged lymph glands, a feeling of not being well or severe headaches. This illness lasts for a few days. Now there are many illnesses that cause these same symptoms, so don't be alarmed every time you get a fever, unless you are engaging in risky behavior.

Asymptomatic Stage or Stage 2 — In this stage, you have no symptoms or signs of disease. You look and feel healthy. This stage can last from several months to several years. We know some people who became ill within two months of infection, and some people who are still healthy after several years.

We know the virus was present in this country by the mid-1970s from blood taken from a number of homosexual men in San Francisco. At that time there was no AIDS epidemic, and there was no test for the AIDS virus. The blood was being tested for different reasons, and it was stored for future testing. After the tests for AIDS were developed in 1985, the blood was unfrozen and tested. A number of men were identified as being HIV infected.

This group of men have been followed very carefully. Some of those men are still alive, 17 years later. Every year the percentage of men still alive has declined, but it is possible that you can have the virus and not die for 17 years, perhaps longer. Scientists and physicians do not know why some people stay healthier longer. We wish we did.

During this asymptomatic time, no one can tell that you are infected, not even a doctor, unless you have an AIDS test to check for the antibodies in your blood. It is important to realize there are no visible clues to tell that you are infected.

Symptomatic Stage or Stage 3 — In this stage several symptoms can be found. They may occur either one at a time or several at once. People in this stage can be very ill and even die without going on to the next and final stage in this whole spectrum of disease. These symptoms include:

- *Weight loss* of more than 10 pounds that is not due to dieting, or is not otherwise explainable.
- In children and adolescents, failure to gain weight while still growing.
- *Unexplained fever*, especially when associated with night sweats that drench the bedding or your night clothes. (If you're certain it's just because of menopause/hot flashes, don't worry!)
- *Swollen glands* in more than one place without other symptoms. Or lymph nodes that are larger than the size of a large walnut. Again many people get enlarged lymph nodes from common infections. Don't panic. If you have any concerns that this may be related to HIV infection, please see your doctor.
- *Shortness of breath*, or difficulty in breathing, particularly during ordinary everyday activities such as walking.
- *Diarrhea*, loose or watery stools several times a day for weeks at a time.
- White cottage-cheeselike coating of the tongue or back of the throat called *thrush*. In healthy people, thrush after infancy is very unusual, although it can occur in diabetics or people taking antibiotics.
- *Persistent fatigue* that doesn't go away, even if you are getting enough sleep and are not under stress.

- *Shingles*, an infection of the skin caused by the same virus that causes chicken pox, herpes zoster. The chicken pox virus stays dormant in the nerves of someone who has previously had chicken pox. Under certain circumstances, for example, when your immune system is not working well, the virus comes to life again, causing a severe skin rash. Not everyone who gets shingles is HIV infected, but many HIV-positive people get shingles.
- *Vaginal yeast infections* that keep coming back, are difficult to treat and are unusually severe.
- *Cervical cancer* can occur in any woman. HIV-positive women are more prone to cervical cancers.

Full-blown AIDS or Stage 4 — By now the immune system is so depleted of T-helper cells that unusual illnesses take the opportunity to invade the body of the HIV-infected individual. These are called opportunistic infections. Some of these illnesses I had never heard of while I was in medical school. And some I even find hard to pronounce now. I list them here for your information:

- *Pneumocystis carinii pneumonia (PCP)* — an infection of the lung causing difficulty with breathing and death if untreated.
- *Isospora Bella* — an infection causing severe diarrhea that is usually easy to treat if diagnosed.
- *Cryptosporidiosis* — an infection causing diarrhea up to 24 times a day. We have no treatment at present for this disease.
- *Toxoplasmosis* — an infection, usually found in the brain, that can cause confusion, coma, death. It can also be in the eyes, heart or liver. Tennis great Arthur Ashe had toxoplasmosis.
- *Cytomegalo virus* — a virus which can cause pneumonia, blindness and problems with the digestive tract.

- *Esophageal candidiasis* — a fungal infection causing pain when eating.
- *Cryptococcus* — an infection in the brain.
- *Microbacterium avium intracellulare* — intracellular infection causing fever and weight loss.
- Cancers such as Kaposi's sarcoma (KS) and unusual lymphomas often occur in people with full-blown AIDS.

Unfortunately, these are not just multisyllabic words that sound serious — they are diseases that destroy lives.

A patient of mine died recently with blindness in one eye due to cytomegalo virus; partial deafness due to drugs we'd used to treat a life-threatening infection; Kaposi's sarcoma in his leg, causing him difficulty in walking, and in his lungs, causing him difficulty in breathing; a rare form of tuberculosis for which he was on four different kinds of medicines, which made him nauseous; a bleeding tendency caused by his inability to produce platelets which are needed to stop bleeding; a seizure disorder and an irregular heartbeat.

This is a horrendous disease for a patient to have and a nightmare for a doctor to treat.

There is no cure for AIDS, but many of the infections that people with AIDS get, such as PCP, can now be treated or even prevented.

When I first started seeing AIDS patients in 1985, we had many patients with PCP. And many of them died. The second woman I ever treated with AIDS died of PCP within two weeks of our making a diagnosis. Now if we know a person is HIV infected, we can prevent the occurrence of PCP by simply giving the proper medication. And if PCP is diagnosed, we are much better at treating it. No one in the last several years of my practice has died of PCP.

We also know how to delay the progression of AIDS with drugs such as AZT, also known as Retrovir or Zidovudine.

Two similar drugs, DDI and DDC, were approved for use later. Patients can live much longer and healthier lives now compared to a few years ago, if they are diagnosed early. AIDS can be treated as a chronic disease that ultimately results in death, rather than as an instant death sentence. However, I must stress there is no vaccine yet to prevent the spread of the virus nor cure for AIDS.

History Of HIV In the United States

I saw my first case of HIV disease in 1982 while I was a resident, but I didn't know it at the time. It was only years later that I would be able to name this disease.

This man had large lymph nodes in his neck, under his arm and in his groin. I had never seen anything like it nor had any of the residents I worked with. Brian was a very handsome body-builder who was frightened by his symptoms.

I discussed his case with a consultant who asked me if Brian was homosexual. I didn't understand what sexual orientation had to do with anything and asked him why he wanted to know. He said something about a "new gay man's disease."

Well, I thought, my patient wasn't gay. He wasn't effeminate, he didn't speak in the way I associated with other gay men and he was a macho body builder.

Knowing how to ask someone if he was homosexual was not something I had been taught to do, and so I never did ask Brian and never diagnosed what was wrong with him. I left my residency program a few weeks later still without having made a diagnosis on him. Even if I had suspected that this was the new gay man's disease, there was no way to confirm that diagnosis at the time. There was no test prior to 1985 to help us identify who was infected.

In retrospect, I am sure Brian knew the magnitude if not the name of his disease before I did. I have learned a lot about characterizing people and about this disease since then.

When a good friend of mine died of AIDS in 1983, it took me a long time to understand the cause of her death. In 1982 she was involved in a traffic accident and needed a blood transfusion. She never was well after that, having one strange illness after another, including severe cold sores, thrush and an unusual lack of energy. We thought she had leukemia. It wasn't until three years later that I understood what disease had killed her.

No one knows exactly how the Human Immunodeficiency Virus originated. The virus was presumably introduced into the United States in the 1970s, and AIDS was first recognized clinically in 1981. Although no one knows whether this is a new disease, or where it came from, some people suggest the virus was in Africa at least ten years before it came to the United States. We don't know whether the virus was present in humans before the first documented evidence. It may have been present first in animals and then transmitted to humans.

One theory holds that this virus may have entered the United States in 1976, perhaps during the Bicentennial celebrations in New York City when thousands of people from around the world took part in the festivities.

It wasn't until June 5, 1981, that the first symptoms of HIV infection in the United States were reported by the Centers for Disease Control (CDC). The report stated that five young men, all sexually active homosexuals, were treated for a very rare pneumonia in Los Angeles. This rare pneumonia was PCP. One month later, the Centers for Disease Control reported that Kaposi's sarcoma, a very rare cancer previously found only in men over the age of 60, had been diagnosed in 26 homosexual men. Only one woman was diagnosed with AIDS that year.

We didn't realize it then, but from this point on the world would never be the same. Sex would never be the same.

One year later, on July 9, 1982, the CDC reported several opportunistic infections, including PCP, Kaposi's sarcoma and oral thrush, among 34 Haitians residing in the United States. On July 16, 1982, the CDC reported three cases of PCP among three heterosexual males with hemophilia, none of whom used intravenous drugs. At the same time, the CDC indicated there was evidence that what was then called a deficiency syndrome might be transmitted through blood products.

This theory was to be confirmed within the year. At the same time, patients such as Haitians and infants — with none of the known risk factors of homosexuality and IV drug use — were being diagnosed.

In 1983 both Robert Gallo from the National Cancer Institute of the United States and Luc Montagnier, of the Pasteur Institute of France, independently discovered the virus that eventually would be called HIV. Gallo called it Human T Lymphtropic Virus Type 3 (HTLV III), and Montagnier called it Lymphadenopathy Associated Virus (LAV).

In the next few years the facts about HIV and AIDS became clear, and the need to educate people became compelling. In an effort to educate the general public, the U.S. Surgeon General mailed an informational brochure on AIDS to every household in the country on May 6, 1988. The brochure, titled "Understanding AIDS," outlined transmission patterns for HIV, discussed testing and emphasized the need for psychosocial support for those infected with the virus.

By that time, many of us in the healthcare field felt the same urgency and began to discuss abstinence, safer sex and the dangers of IV drug use with anyone who would listen. But most people felt this was not their disease, and they did little or nothing to change their lifestyle.

In the 1990s, though most people with HIV in the United States are gay and bisexual men, the disease is increasingly a disease of the young and the heterosexual, with the rate of infection in women expanding at an alarming pace.

AFRAIDS (Acute Fear Regarding AIDS)

Some people have a tremendous, often irrational, fear of AIDS. They don't even want to be in the same room with a person who is HIV infected for fear of becoming infected themselves. We call this *"AFRAIDS."*

The good news about AIDS and HIV is that if we take reasonable precautions to protect ourselves from this disease, there is no need to panic.

The AIDS virus, fortunately, does not spread through day-to-day casual contact. We are really fortunate because the HIV cannot survive in air, in water or on things people touch, unlike some other viruses like influenza or measles. This virus survives only in the blood and some body fluids of infected people. Even if infected people sneeze or cough, you aren't in danger of getting the virus from them because you don't take any of their fluids into your body.

I've taken care of many HIV-infected people. I touch them, I hug them, I examine them, I hold their hands. I've seen enough people die of this disease to know that I don't want to get it. And I'm not going to take any chances. I am tested regularly and, not surprisingly, I've remained negative.

Anyone can be infected without knowing it. So I assume that everyone has HIV, and I'm careful with everyone. By that I mean I wear gloves when I'm dealing with the blood or body fluids of any patient. And I'm extremely careful not to stick myself with a needle that I have used on any patient. In the healthcare profession, we call this practicing "universal precautions," assuming that everyone we work with is infected with HIV or another contagious disease.

My methods to protect myself from infection do not prevent me from showing compassion and concern for people with HIV. You cannot get this virus by touching or hugging someone.

Household members of people with AIDS have been tested in many studies and there has been no evidence of spread to any family or household members or close contacts, except to needle-sharing partners or sex partners of infected people.

You can't catch this virus by doing everyday things like going to school, shopping and trying on clothes in a department store. You cannot get AIDS from sitting next to someone in school who has the virus, using the toilet, drinking from the same water fountain, using the telephone or visiting someone who has AIDS. You cannot get this virus from swimming in a pool, standing in a crowd or by being bitten by a mosquito.

You can only get this virus from sex or from blood, including blood-contaminated needles.

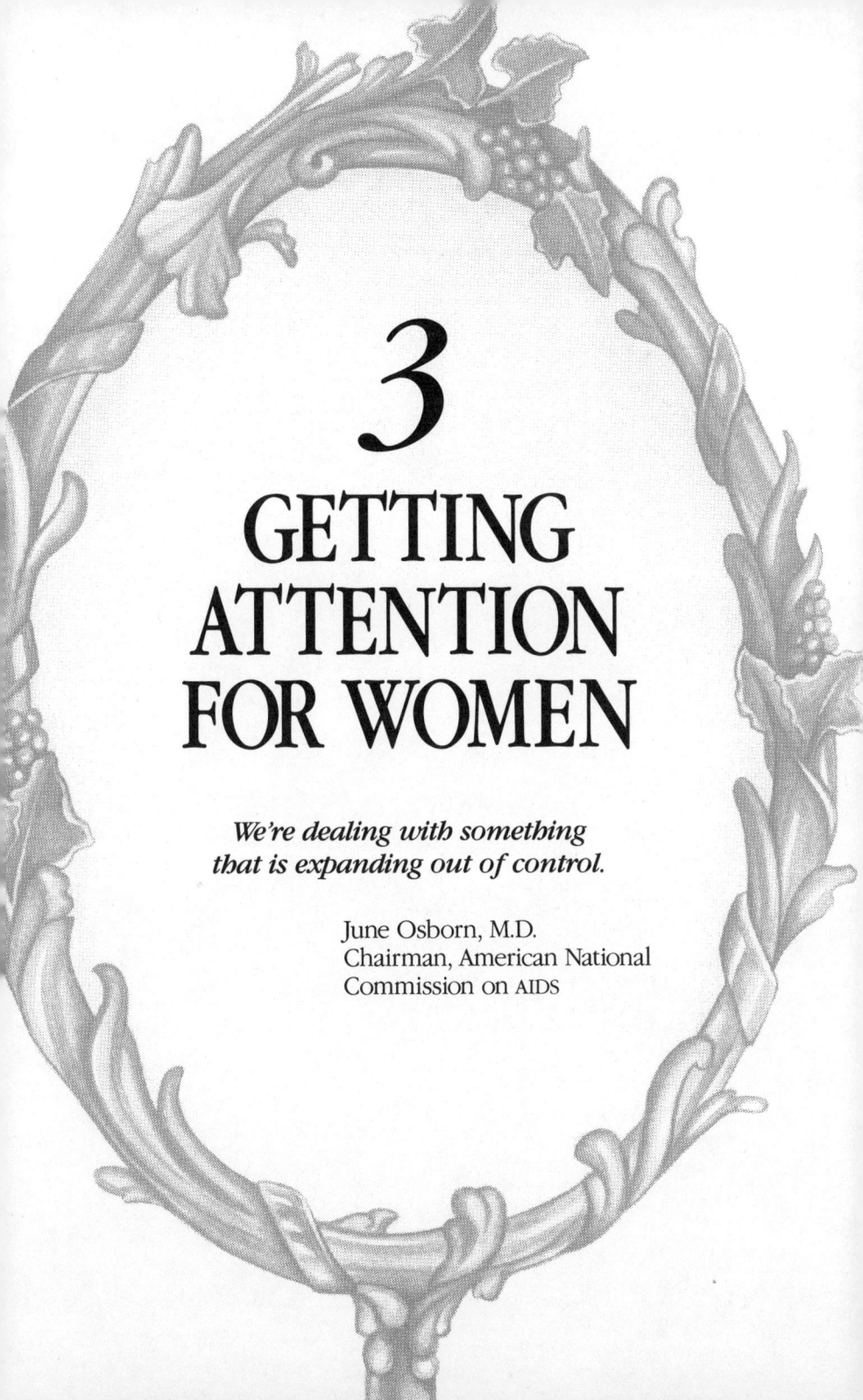

3
GETTING ATTENTION FOR WOMEN

We're dealing with something that is expanding out of control.

June Osborn, M.D.
Chairman, American National
Commission on AIDS

*P*erhaps we shouldn't be surprised that women are still not getting their fair share of attention on AIDS issues from medical and research institutes. AIDS first entered our awareness in the United States chiefly as a disease of gay men. By 1990, however, the statistics began shifting rapidly and now we know AIDS is an equal opportunity disease. We should all be on the rooftops shouting for equal research funds and medical benefits.

At least three million women in the world will die of AIDS during the decade of the '90s. Seventy-five percent of them will have been infected simply by having a sexual relationship with an infected man. Some will be infected by loving husbands and committed partners, men they trusted enough to have unprotected sex with.

Everyday these numbers become outdated. Everyday we learn more about this disease. And everyday more people are infected and more people die. The truth is, while close watch is kept on the numbers of reported AIDS cases, there is an unknown number of deaths, especially those of women, which go unreported as AIDS related.

How can this be? The fact is that the Centers for Disease Control in Atlanta, which is the national "scorekeeper" of AIDS occurrences, is currently using a definition for AIDS that excludes many women who actually have the disease.

AIDS is diagnosed only when certain opportunistic diseases occur among HIV-infected individuals. That definition does not include any of the gynecological conditions so often present in women with AIDS, such as cervical cancer. These conditions are not uncommon in healthy women, but they do prove deadly for a woman infected with HIV.

The CDC in May 1992 postponed for the third time changing the AIDS definition. Some estimate that if the definition changes, the number of reported AIDS cases in this country will more than double, rising from an estimated 200,000 to 440,000. Many of those cases would be women.

While changing the definition is important in keeping track of the number of people dying from this disease, it's even more critical to women who do not qualify for Social Security and other benefits unless the diagnosis of AIDS is made based on the current definition.

This means a woman with AIDS too sick to support herself may not get the financial assistance she desperately needs if she is diagnosed as just a cervical cancer case.

We don't really know how many people are infected with HIV. There is no law requiring those who have been tested and know they are infected to be reported to the CDC or public health departments. And many more people haven't been tested, so they don't know that they are infected and possibly spreading the disease to others. The estimates of 1.5 million infected people in this country are based on complicated epidemiological formulas.

One of the most important things to remember is the treacherous time factor. People diagnosed with AIDS today could have been infected 10 or more years ago. That means a young woman who contracted the virus having her first sexual relationship with her high school sweetheart in 1978 could be coming to the doctor's office now for AIDS-related symptoms.

As with so many other healthcare issues that concern women, little is known about AIDS and how it specifically affects women. Even though it still is primarily a disease that kills men, and most of the research to date on this disease and its possible treatments has been focused on men, the rapid rise in the rate of infection in women means it is imperative to focus attention on women now.

Even the media has focused primarily on the men with the disease, starting with stars like Rock Hudson, who first made it okay to talk about AIDS. Then Magic Johnson hit home with men — young and old — who began to realize that this disease can be transmitted through casual sex between men and women. Actually I don't think Magic is conveying the whole message. He still looks so healthy, it looks as if AIDS is no big deal. And what about all those women he had sex with? Surely some of them got AIDS from that encounter. Don't they count?

When tennis star Arthur Ashe came forward with the news that he had been infected with HIV by a blood transfusion, it frightened thousands of people who had also had blood transfusions in the years prior to testing of donated blood for HIV. If these people went out for HIV tests now and came up positive, at least they could receive life-prolonging medical help and notify their sexual partners past and present.

Certainly celebrities are doing a great amount of good with their admissions, but it's outrageous to think we had to wait for a movie or sports star or Elizabeth Glaser at the Democratic National Convention to announce *she* has

AIDS before the women of this country woke up to the danger of this epidemic. It's as if everything has to have some kind of entertainment value before it's publicized enough for people to really understand the risks they face. And believe me, there's no connection whatsoever between AIDS and entertainment.

What We Know About Women And HIV/AIDS

Here's what we do know about women with HIV disease and AIDS:

Transmission

A woman is 12 times more likely to be infected by a man than the man is likely to be infected by his female partner. While we're not sure why this is, we believe it's because the woman's vagina may have tiny tears that allow the HIV-infected semen to enter her body. Also if no condom is used, the semen stays in her vagina and cervix long after the man's penis has withdrawn, offering more time for infection to occur. A woman's reproductive organs were designed to hold semen. Unless the man's penis has a cut or sore, he is less likely to get infected vaginal secretions into his body.

Ironically, while evidence shows that men are much more efficient at spreading HIV disease, women have often been referred to as "vectors" in this epidemic, meaning that they were a means of transmitting the virus to men and their babies. And the old double standards regarding sex have been applied to this disease, leaving the infected woman with a stigma not shared by her male counterpart.

Back to the example of Magic Johnson. He admits to having 2,000 sex partners, and he's called sexually active. If a woman admits to more than a few partners, she's called promiscuous, a slut, a loose woman or a whore.

Diagnosis: Women Die Faster

Women aren't being diagnosed as early as men and are thus losing out on earlier life-prolonging treatments. It appears that with early diagnosis they have the same life expectancy as HIV-infected men.

Gynecological infections such as pelvic inflammatory disease, yeast infections and cervical cancer can be the first signs of HIV disease in women. It's estimated that between 50 and 65 percent of HIV-positive women die from these ailments, but they won't be counted as AIDS-related deaths because the definition of an AIDS case does not include any gynecological infections. That may change as powerful organizations, such as the American Medical Association and the Center for Women Policy Studies lobby for the AIDS definition to be broadened.

Evidence suggests that by the time a woman is diagnosed with AIDS, she'll die four to six times faster than a man. All too often, a woman isn't diagnosed until she gets pregnant, her baby is born HIV infected or she is hospitalized with an opportunistic disease associated with the onset of AIDS. If a man walks into a doctor's office complaining of night sweats and swollen glands, a doctor will more likely test him for the AIDS virus. If a woman walks in with similar symptoms, she's more apt to be told not to worry, this disease isn't about women.

Doctors May Not
Recognize AIDS In Women

One of the first women I saw with AIDS had been placed in an eating disorder unit for treatment of what doctors thought was anorexia. Christine had lost 40 pounds over a few months, and her doctors couldn't find anything else wrong with her. She didn't have an appetite, and she couldn't eat.

While in this specialized unit, Christine began to have fevers and coughing. An X ray showed there was something else wrong with her. Christine's doctor asked me to consult on the case because he suspected pneumocystis carinii pneumonia (PCP), a rare lung disease that usually signals the onset of AIDS.

By the time I saw Christine and diagnosed AIDS, it was too late to help her. She died a few weeks later.

The fact that Christine's doctors didn't think to test her for HIV isn't unusual. I've had many patients tell me that other doctors would not test them even when they asked. Thankfully most of these women breathe a sigh of relief when I do the test and it comes back negative. Unfortunately a growing number of them are finding out they are HIV infected.

Louise is another patient of mine. She is in her early 40s and believes she acquired the virus from a man she met in August 1989, while she was separated from her husband.

That fall, she first began to notice things weren't right with her body. "A friend was giving me a massage, and he found swollen lymph glands in my neck," she recalled. "I pointed them out to my doctor who thought the swelling was related to an accident I'd had a few weeks before. But within two months, I lost 25 pounds. That was in December. In February I again talked with my doctor and said something was wrong. I had night sweats, no appetite, diarrhea and swollen glands.

"When I asked my doctor to test me for AIDS, he said I was white and female, that it wouldn't happen to me," Louise said. It wasn't until August, a year after the time she suspects she was infected, that the doctor finally ran the AIDS test.

"He cried when he told me it was positive, but I could only feel anger at him," Louise said. "He should have been trained to take care of me. If you find out that you are HIV infected, you can change your life that day, but because he didn't test me, a year of my life was wasted. I could have been taking care of myself better had I known I was HIV positive."

Since her diagnosis, Louise has stopped drinking and smoking and is taking care not to stress her body needlessly. There is some evidence to suggest that living a healthy lifestyle will help the body's immune system ward off the AIDS virus longer.

Testing

Nationwide, there are public health departments, clinics and physician offices offering anonymous, sometimes free testing for people who want to know if they're infected. Private physicians can also run the HIV test on their patients. But all too often a woman who looks healthy is not tested by her physician.

Doctors are no different from other people. As long as they have a preconceived notion that they can tell if a person is at risk for having HIV disease simply by knowing her income level and ethnic background, many women will go untested and will live in fear that they may be infected. Women need to be more assertive in demanding that they be tested by their physicians, even if their doctor believes they are not at risk.

Treatment

We have made some progress in extending the lives of people with AIDS, through the development of AZT, DDC and DDI, and other drugs that help ward off the opportunistic infections which used to kill people early in their disease. While we still haven't found a cure for AIDS, we have found ways to manage it more like a chronic illness, treating more effectively the various diseases an HIV-infected person may have. But AZT, as with most other drugs, has not been extensively tested on women. It is being used on women without benefit of knowing whether it reacts differently in females, or whether it will damage the fetus of a pregnant woman.

While the federal government has increased funding for AIDS research considerably, escalating from $216,000 in 1983 to more than $14 billion in 1987, little has been targeted to women. We don't know, for example, the effects of contraceptives, such as birth control pills, the five-year Norplant or IUDs on women with HIV disease. (And yet preventing pregnancy may be of critical importance to a woman who is sick with HIV disease.)

The intrauterine device (IUD) may make an HIV-infected woman more likely to pass the disease on to her partner. She bleeds more heavily during her period, and that makes it easier to infect the male. Also the tail of the device could cause small cuts in the penis during intercourse. The infected woman herself might be more susceptible to other infections such as pelvic inflammatory disease.

We know little about how to care for the pregnant woman who is also carrying the AIDS virus. Usually when a woman is pregnant, we'll try not to give her too many drugs for fear of harming the fetus. With the HIV-infected mother, however, doctors are torn between giving her AZT or withholding the life-prolonging drug for fear of harming the fetus. Little research is available because the drug trials testing AZT originally excluded women. This was done to avoid the possibility of testing a pregnant woman and the unknown effects of the drug on the fetus.

We also don't know much about the potential damage to the fetus when treating the pregnant mother for any of a host of opportunistic infections that may invade her body during the pregnancy.

Education And Prevention

Any educator knows that in order to reach certain groups of people with messages that will motivate them to change, a host of factors must be taken into account. This is true with the message that AIDS is killing women, and that women need to take responsibility for protecting themselves. It sounds like an easy message. But for education to be effective, we have to take into account that we must reach all types of women: The single woman who is struggling to find a way to feed her children, and who may do anything to find some sense of security and comfort in a world filled with doubt and pain. The woman who is trapped in an abusive relationship, where to bring up the subject of using a condom could result in a fatal beating. The woman who feels safe and protected from harm because of the sanctity of marriage. The teenager who thinks she'll live forever.

There is a crying need for AIDS awareness programs aimed at reaching women. They must not only hear the message, they must also be empowered to do whatever is needed to protect themselves.

It's difficult to convince the women I know that they should be concerned about AIDS. I've had women say that they're much more concerned about dying of breast cancer, a disease that strikes one out of nine women each year, or from heart disease — the number one killer of women. If you can't get a woman to have a yearly mammogram to detect breast cancer early, how can you get her to learn to say no to unprotected sex? Or to have an AIDS test done when the fear of a positive result is so awesome?

Others say, "Getting AIDS is just like getting cancer or any other terminal disease. Horrible, yes, but we've all got to die sometime." That type of nonchalance angers me because this disease, unlike cancer, can be prevented. It only takes stopping unprotected sex and sharing dirty needles.

Unless women realize that this disease is going to kill thousands of our sisters, daughters, mothers and friends

— women who had hoped to marry and one day have children, women who wanted to see their children grow up and have children of their own — it will continue to escalate at alarming speed.

Women have only recently begun to lobby Congress for increased research into breast cancer, heart disease, osteoporosis and estrogen replacement therapy. This effort has begun to pay off with the development of the Office of Women's Health Research through the National Institutes of Health (NIH). It is the job of this office to make sure that women are included in clinical research trials conducted by the NIH. Also the NIH is launching a major women's health research initiative that will involve 140,000 women over the next 10 years. Studies will focus on cardiovascular disease, cancer, diet and osteoporosis in women. This is good news.

But research is also needed on women and AIDS. I was lecturing recently before a group of businesswomen, and a woman in the audience asked, "Why should we spend so much money on AIDS when so few women are dying from this disease? That money should go into cancer and heart disease research."

My answer to her was that AIDS is a disease that takes about 10 years to show up in people from the time they are infected. We're just beginning to see the results of what happened 10 years ago. I don't want to wait until 110 million people in this world are infected before we say this disease deserves its share of the research dollars. This is a contagious disease, transmitted from one person to another. The longer we leave it alone to proliferate, the more generations of doctors, lawyers, farmers, mothers and fathers we'll lose.

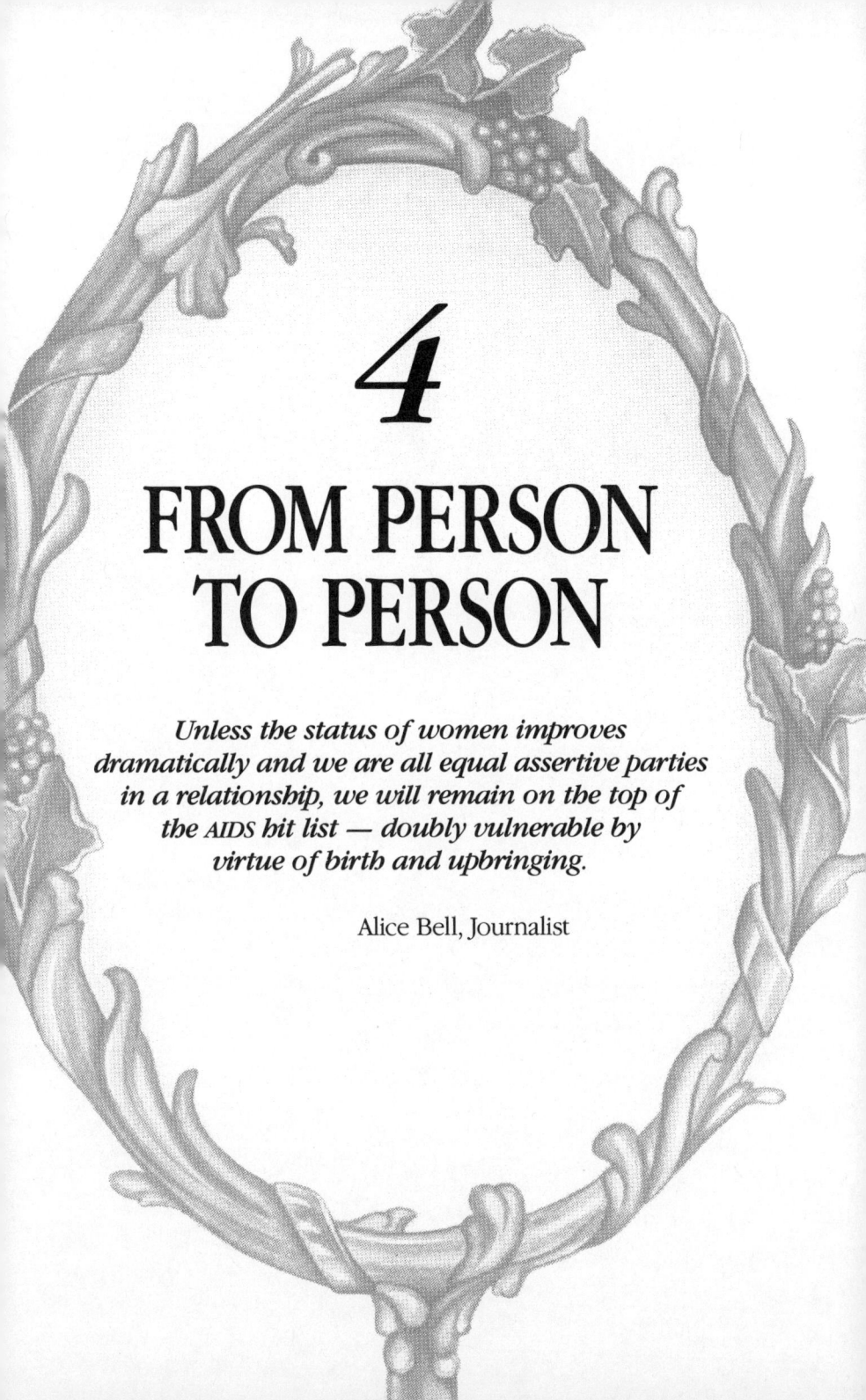

4

FROM PERSON TO PERSON

Unless the status of women improves dramatically and we are all equal assertive parties in a relationship, we will remain on the top of the AIDS hit list — doubly vulnerable by virtue of birth and upbringing.

Alice Bell, Journalist

*T*he AIDS virus is passed from person to person by exchanging body fluids. Body fluids include blood, vaginal secretions and semen. They can be exchanged in ways you may not have considered possible.

Body Fluids

Blood

The AIDS virus is found in blood. You should practice what healthcare workers call universal precautions — act as if everyone is infected when it comes to dealing with someone else's blood. If your skin is intact, there is no real danger of another person's blood entering your body. However, we don't always know if we have hangnails, sores or cuts and so it is prudent to use some kind of barrier to keep someone else's blood from getting on your skin. If blood does get on your skin, promptly wash your hands with soap and water.

Avoid blood contact in the following ways:

- Don't share razors or toothbrushes with someone else. There is a possibility of sharing any blood that may be on them.
- If you are ever in the position of helping someone who is bleeding, make sure you use some type of barrier to prevent the blood from getting on your skin. Towels, clothes, rubber gloves, plastic wrap or whatever is handy can help protect you.
- The AIDS virus is very fragile and dies quickly when in contact with air. More importantly than what you use to clean blood is that you take care to protect your hands, wearing gloves if possible.
- If blood gets on your clothes, wash them in hot soapy water.
- Bathroom facilities should be kept clean. Blood and other body fluids should be flushed down the toilet. If there's a spill, it should be cleaned properly, taking care to protect your hands from coming into contact with the spill. When discarding used tampons or sanitary napkins, please wrap them in tissue to help protect the person cleaning the restroom.
- Don't share needles — not for steroid injections, ear piercing, tattooing, insulin injections, allergy shots or for any other reason. Used needles should be disposed of properly. Just imagine how you'd feel if you picked up a bag of trash and accidentally were stuck by a needle someone had thrown in without thinking about the consequences. Even though the virus dies quickly in the air, there is a slight chance that this needle, if used on an infected person and then thrown away, could infect another.
- The old tradition of being "blood brothers and sisters" is a thing of the past. If you ever catch your children talking about being someone's blood brother, please have a talk with them.

• Don't have sex (either oral or vaginal) when you are a menstruating female if there is any chance you are HIV infected. HIV infected menstrual blood can be very infectious to your partner.

Vaginal Fluids

The virus is found in the vagina and in the vaginal fluids. Having vaginal sex with a woman without a condom is not safe for the male partner since the virus can enter his body through the penis or urethra. Oral sex performed on a woman without a dental dam or piece of rubber latex between her genital area and your mouth is also not safe since the virus may be swallowed or may enter the body through cuts in the mouth. You can also use non-microwavable plastic wrap (doubled over for extra protection) over the female genital areas.

Pre-ejaculate Fluid And Semen

The virus is found in the pre-ejaculate fluid as well as in the semen. Thus a condom should be worn during any sexual activity, including oral, vaginal or rectal sex, to prevent these fluids from touching any part of a partner's body.

Saliva

The virus can be found in the saliva in very small quantities. We do not know of a single case where kissing was the way the virus was spread. You can't get it by drinking out of the same glass or sharing eating utensils.

Mother To Baby

An HIV-positive mother has about a 30 percent chance of infecting her unborn baby. Unfortunately, the virus has also been found in breast milk, and a few babies have been infected while nursing from their mother.

How Safe Is Safe?
How Risky Is Risky?

Most adults are sexually active. The average number of sex partners an American has during his or her adult life is seven. Obviously, it's impossible to tell adults to stop having sex. But there are ways of protecting yourself from HIV disease while still enjoying a sexual relationship. Some sexual activities have a very low risk and others are extremely risky. Here are some guidelines.

Assess Your Risk

No-Risk Sex — Celibacy.

Ultra-Safe Sex — Sex without touching, such as telephone sex, fantasizing about sex, reading or watching pornography. It is said that the brain is the largest sex organ and can create images and use words to arouse, delight and satisfy.

Safe Sex — Dry sex, with no exchange of body fluids, including caressing, touching, hugging, self-masturbation, dry kissing and massaging nongenital areas of the body, such as the toes, knees, ears, eyes, neck and elbows; petting, fully clothed, partially clothed or totally undressed.

Low Risk — Wet, deep or French kissing, as long as you don't kiss if you or your partner has sores, or if you have not vigorously brushed your teeth or dental flossed, causing bleeding. Using a condom for oral, vaginal or anal sex with a person you know is not infected. Mutual masturbation if you have no cuts on your hands and if vaginal fluid or semen does not get on the partner's body.

High Risk — Using a condom for oral, vaginal or anal sex with a partner who is at high risk of being HIV infected. Rimming or oral-anal contact. Watersports, urinating into the vagina or the rectum. Fisting (inserting a hand or fist into the rectum or vagina). Sharing sex toys such as dildos and vibrators unless they are properly cleaned before and after each use.

Suicidal Sex — Having unprotected sex with a stranger or with a partner who is at high risk of being infected or is infected.

The riskiest sexual activity of all is anal (or rectal) sex. Some women have anal sex in order to maintain their virginity, some enjoy this type of sexual activity and others engage in it to prevent pregnancy. This is a common form of birth control in Third World countries.

Female partners of HIV-positive men who engage in anal sex are two to three times more likely to acquire the virus than females who don't practice anal intercourse. What makes this so risky is that the walls of the rectum are fragile and easily torn, allowing blood and semen to pass from one person to another.

IV Drug Use And AIDS

If you or someone you have a relationship with has ever engaged in IV drug use, you should know that 30 percent of all AIDS cases reported in the United States have involved IV drug users.

This is important to note since, as in Sherry's story, you may be involved with someone who long ago shared a needle with an HIV-infected person. As of May 1991, at least 3,673 women were known to have contracted AIDS through a sexual relationship with an infected IV drug user. These were women of all ages and economic levels, although most were of childbearing age and economically deprived. Most were not aware of or didn't want to know about their partner's history of IV drug use.

If you or your partner is addicted to drugs or alcohol, please seek treatment. If you or your sex partner shoot drugs, insist on safer sex practices every time you have sex to protect both of you from infection.

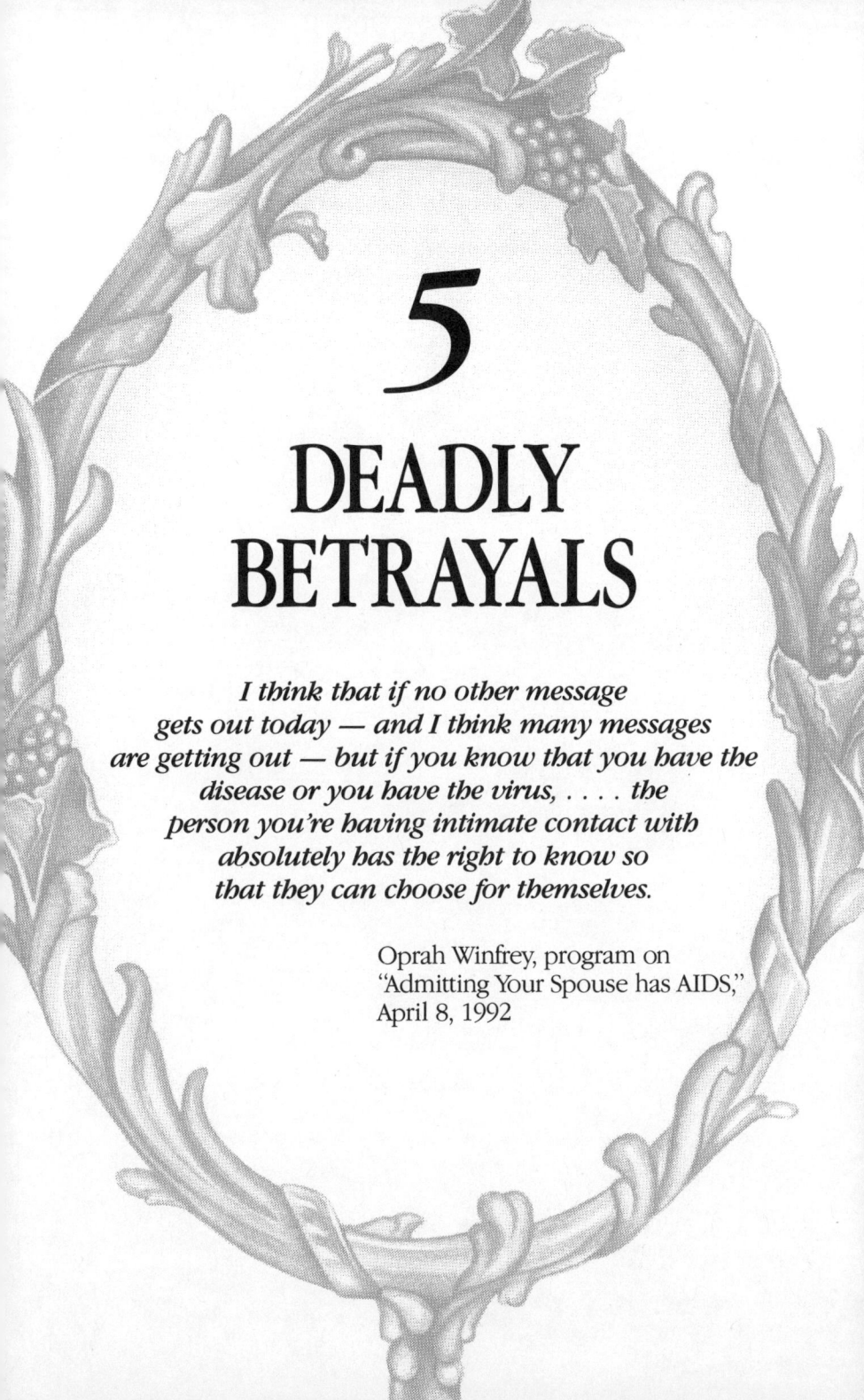

5

DEADLY BETRAYALS

*I think that if no other message
gets out today — and I think many messages
are getting out — but if you know that you have the
disease or you have the virus, ... the
person you're having intimate contact with
absolutely has the right to know so
that they can choose for themselves.*

Oprah Winfrey, program on
"Admitting Your Spouse has AIDS,"
April 8, 1992

*I*s marriage safe? We'd all like to think so, but the answer to that important question is, maybe not. If you think this epidemic won't affect you because you're in a mutually faithful relationship with an uninfected partner, remember: Even though most people believe in and want monogamy, more than 60 percent of married men and 40 percent of married women have extramarital affairs.

Marriage and commitment don't always stop the chemical attraction or electrical charge that sometimes occurs between a man and a woman. Sometimes an affair lasts one night, sometimes it can continue for many years. Sometimes it's the woman who has the affair, sometimes it's the man. Older men tend to prefer to have affairs with younger, single women. Women tend to have liaisons with older married men.

In *The Hite Report*, it was estimated that 70 percent of women married for more than five years, and 72 percent of men married for more than two years, have sex outside of their marriage. These are grave statistics to contemplate when you're thinking about your chances of becoming infected with HIV. Apparently very few married people are immune to having affairs.

Often these marriages have respect, trust and love, and the affairs are not a result of insensitivity or lack of moral conscience. The affair more often than not is only about sex. Many wives are content to turn their heads, ignoring their husbands' "little affairs."

I have friends, colleagues, family members and patients who have had or are having affairs. And some marriages have survived in spite of, or even because of, the infidelity.

If affairs are common, so is denial about affairs. According to *The Hite Report*, 79 percent of women didn't believe their husbands were having affairs, even though only 28 percent of men married for more than two years were still monogamous. Affairs are usually characterized by secretiveness and dishonesty.

Now, more than ever, honesty is essential in a loving relationship. Some counselors in the past might have advised against confessing an affair out of the belief that what the partner doesn't know won't hurt them. Today that way of thinking could cost a life.

Sometimes my female patients confide their fears to me that their husbands or lovers may be having affairs. While finding out that your lover was unfaithful may be emotionally devastating, it's better to know so that you can take the steps necessary to protect yourself from a possible infection.

Even though statistics indicate extramarital affairs are not unusual, society judges those who have them harshly, which makes it even more difficult for partners to discuss these situations honestly. While sexual freedom and openness work for some, the topic of sex is still uncomfortable for many women to discuss, even in the marriage bed. And the romance myth dies hard. Longing to believe they have fairy tale marriages with perfect partners prevents wives from asking husbands about his affairs and certainly makes women reluctant to confess any indiscretion they may have committed themselves. Because we want to live in that safe bubble of belief, our affairs are shrouded in guilt, shame, embarrassment, resentment, bitterness and pain.

The need to avoid these unpleasant emotions keeps us from talking about sexual relationships which might bring the AIDS virus into the marriage.

Your Relationship Self-Evaluation

If you are in a marriage or other committed relationship and wonder about your safety, I suggest you ask yourself these questions:

- Is your life more important than your relationship?
- Are you prepared to take the necessary steps to protect yourself, even if that could possibly jeopardize your relationship?
- Is your relationship more important than the affair?
- Is your relationship strong enough to weather the affair if your partner is willing to work it out with you?

What To Ask Your Partner

Once you know these answers, I would encourage you to talk to your partner, sharing with him your fears, not only about his suspected affair, but also about your contracting a disease from him.

You could say, "I'd like you to be honest with me about whether you are having an affair. I hope the answer is no, but, more importantly, I hope you'll answer me truthfully. If the answer is yes, we'll need to look at our relationship carefully, but it's not necessarily the end of our life together.

"However, if you lie to me, and I find out later, I think that might be the end of our relationship."

If your lover admits to having sex outside your relationship, even an occasional one-night stand, here are some of the steps to take to protect yourself from possible infection.

- There's little point in asking about the sexual history of the other person involved. You'll probably never know if that person is infected or not.
- Whether or not safer sex was practiced, I suggest testing. If the affair was over more than six months ago, have your partner and yourself tested. If he won't be tested, then either abstain from having sex with him or use condoms until a test is taken.
- If the affair ended less than six months ago, ask him to be tested now, and again six months after the last sexual encounter in that affair.
- If you think he is still having the affair or will have affairs in the future, you should either abstain from having sex with him, or at least insist on using condoms for every sexual encounter.

I have a friend who is in her early 50s. Gloria married a very wealthy man whom she loved dearly. Six months into the marriage, he began drinking heavily and staying out all night. When she confronted him, he refused to say whether or not he was having sex outside their marriage. Not knowing what risk he was taking, Gloria decided that her life was more valuable than being a rich man's wife. She left him. She said it almost broke her heart, but she knew she had to do it.

"When it came right down to the tough choice between love and money on one hand and my life on the other, I chose life," Gloria said.

If You Are Having An Affair

On the other hand, some women also tell me they either had or are having an affair outside their committed relationship and wonder if, because of the AIDS epidemic, they should tell their partner.

If you're one of these women, here's what I suggest:

- Examine your committed relationship, and for a moment, put aside the AIDS epidemic. Is your relationship worth having and if so, are you willing to be honest with your partner about the affair, so that you can begin rebuilding the relationship? Often this process will take the help of a marriage counselor.
- If the answer is no, then ask yourself why you are staying in this relationship. Again you may need the help of a counselor.
- Now add AIDS into the equation. If the affair was more than six months ago, you can be tested to see if you were infected. If the results are negative, then you and your partner are safe from the AIDS virus.
- If the affair was less than six months ago, you should be tested and use condoms until you're retested six months after your last sexual encounter in the affair.
- If you do test positive, both of your partners should be told and tested.

If you or your partner have confessed to an affair, and have forgiven each other, your relationship can go on with the pain of that affair fading as time passes. However, from a medical point of view, forgiveness won't make AIDS go away.

Heterosexual affairs aren't the only game in town. Men and women have affairs, women have affairs with women and men have affairs with men. Eleven percent of men say they prefer sex with another man, and six percent of men surveyed in *The Hite Report* have sex with men *and* women. Many bisexual men are married and have homosexual relationships as well.

Romance In The Park

Dan was a happily married university professor who enjoyed anonymous sex with a man he would meet in a park on Sundays. He came to me for testing and the results came back showing that he was infected with HIV. He immediately told his wife and they began to use condoms to protect her from possible infection. The Sunday afternoon affair stopped. The professor and his wife began intensive marital counseling. They're still married today, but I wonder how she deals with the emotional consequences of his having had an affair with another man. She is fortunate she wasn't infected by her husband, yet she still has the devastating problem of dealing with his terminal illness.

I Only Do It With Married Men

Curtis was an HIV-infected patient who came for treatment for recently diagnosed syphilis. Of course, it stands to reason that if he got syphilis, he was not practicing safer sex with use of a condom. If Curtis had contracted syphilis from his partner, then he may, in turn, have infected that person with HIV during the same encounter.

When I asked Curtis about practicing safer sex, he said he didn't think it was necessary since he "only did it with married men." And he didn't think he could get anything from married men. It didn't concern Curtis what he could *give* them.

I was disgusted and horrified. Curtis had no concept of responsibility and didn't care if he was infecting other men. I couldn't get him to show any concern during that office visit. All I could do was warn him that it was a felony to have sex without telling his partner that he was HIV infected.

I was amazed that Curtis trusted that married men wouldn't give him anything — to be so naive when he was having sex with married men himself. And I find it unimaginable for married men to have unsafe sex with other men and then go back to their wives. But I'm told it happens frequently.

I still shake with anger when I think of Curtis. Who knows how many men he infected and how many of those men have infected their wives?

Curtis came to me several weeks later because of a painful skin condition. I had a very hard time trying to be a compassionate doctor in relieving his pain. Because of this inner conflict, I made a decision not to be his physician any longer. Curtis is the only patient I've ever discharged from my practice because I was unable to muster any compassion for him. I believe he is still alive, probably still having unsafe sex — only with married men.

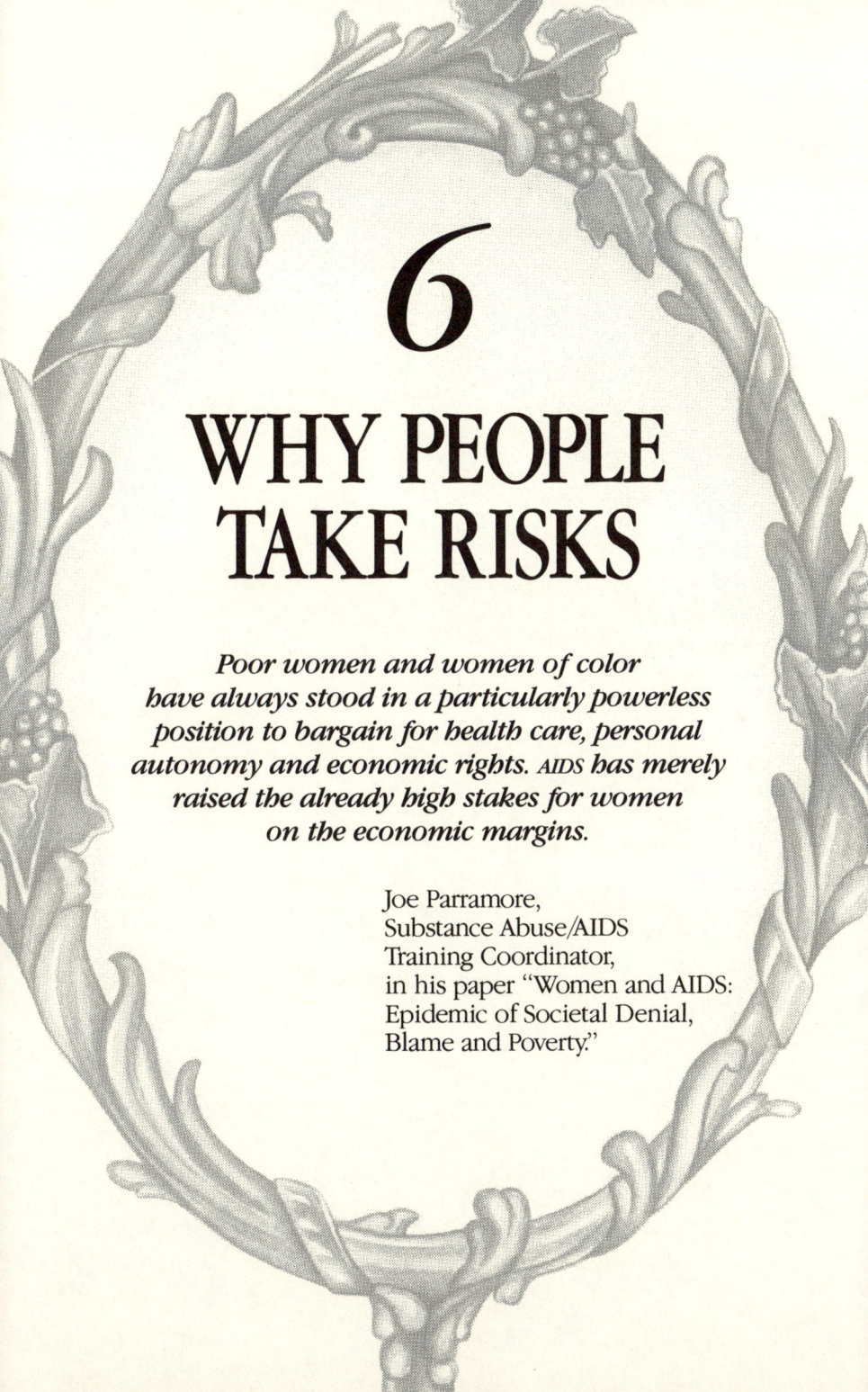

6

WHY PEOPLE TAKE RISKS

*Poor women and women of color
have always stood in a particularly powerless
position to bargain for health care, personal
autonomy and economic rights. AIDS has merely
raised the already high stakes for women
on the economic margins.*

Joe Parramore,
Substance Abuse/AIDS
Training Coordinator,
in his paper "Women and AIDS:
Epidemic of Societal Denial,
Blame and Poverty."

*P*amela is young, pretty, intelligent and faces being HIV positive for the rest of her life. She was probably infected at about the age of 23 by one of her three sex partners. She appears to hold no grudges — in fact, she never refers to how or why she became infected.

Pamela was referred to me by a psychologist who was concerned about her isolation. She had recently been diagnosed and was terrified that she might pass the virus on to someone else.

A college student, Pamela had stopped seeing any of her friends because a classmate had casually taken a sip of her Coke during lunch. She had been told not to share eating utensils with anyone and was afraid she would inadvertently infect her friends.

It took a few office visits with me to convince Pamela that the virus was not casually spread. Eventually she started seeing her friends again. Her parents knew of her diagnosis, and one day she found the strength to share it with a friend, who to her great relief, not only didn't reject her but became a great supporter.

Slowly life became more normal and a few months ago, Pamela celebrated her college graduation. She's always cheerful, is convinced that she's going to "lick this disease," and I hope and pray that she does.

Pamela met a wonderful young man, whom she dated for a while before telling him she was HIV infected. His response was fantastic. He said he wanted to meet me and to learn more about the disease. Pamela and Frank were not yet sexually active, and she swore to me she never would become involved in that way.

"No sex seems safe enough. I couldn't bear the thought of passing this virus on to anyone else, least of all to a man I really care about," she said.

Their friendship has grown into a deep love, and recently, they came to see me again, to hear from me in great detail about safer sex.

Frank looked me straight in the eye and said, "Dr. Sack, I love Pamela, and I want to marry her. I'm going to have sex with her, even if I'm risking my life. None of us know when we're going to die and I certainly don't want to. Teach me how to make love to her as safely as possible."

I cried after they left my office. They are two young people in love, and who knows what their future will be. They will probably marry but have at this point definitely decided against children.

Understanding Human Behavior

What I've learned as a physician is that people don't only have sex with another person because they love and care for that person. Sometimes they have sex with people they hate or fear. Sometimes they have sex out of insecurity, or a need to control, or out of fear of rejection or abandonment.

I am not a sex therapist, but as a family practice physician, I've had to understand sexual behavior so I could teach people how to protect themselves against AIDS. Doctors and others in a position to help prevent AIDS truly don't understand enough about human sexuality. Doctors don't learn enough about it in medical school, nor do teachers in educational degree programs, nor clergy in theological seminaries. Unfortunately neither parents nor politicians are knowledgeable about AIDS either.

In her executive summary, America Living With AIDS, June Osborn, chairman of the National Commission on AIDS, made many recommendations. One was to remove governmental restrictions imposed on the use of funds for certain types of AIDS education, service and research. These restrictions are thought to impede the fight against HIV disease.

"Research into sexual and drug using behaviors must be conducted and evaluated," the commission report stated.

While scientists are struggling to find cures and vaccines for AIDS, we need to struggle to understand human sexuality so we can learn to change risky behaviors. No matter what scientists learn, it still comes down to a matter of personal choice.

Are You Choosing Health?

It has been common knowledge for years that cigarette smoking causes lung cancer, wearing a seatbelt prevents deaths in auto accidents, reducing fat and cholesterol in our diets prevents heart disease. Yet how many of us readily change our lifestyle to adapt to new health rules?

Now, faced with an epidemic requiring us to change sexual behavior, the challenge seems even more difficult. Nevertheless, we need to try to live with heightened consciousness in this, the most personal level of life, if we are to slow down or stop the spread of AIDS.

Love

When you're happy and in love with someone, it's hard to believe your loved one might harbor a killer disease.

When my patients tell me they are madly in love and having wonderful sex, I don't like to burst their bubble and talk to them about AIDS and other sexually transmitted diseases — yet I must.

Having sex with someone you know, love and trust feels safe, but it may not be. For some people who are deeply in love, like Pamela's boyfriend, Frank, the act of making love is somehow more important than protecting themselves from disease. I wish they could be satisfied with love without sex.

I talk about AIDS to everybody. Recently, Maxine, a 60-year-old patient of mine, told me she was in love and having sex again for the first time in many years. She was thrilled. She had been so depressed and now she was having the time of her life.

I considered not talking to her about AIDS, but this virus can infect anyone — no matter how old or how much in love they are. At first, Maxine was shocked. How could AIDS possibly affect her life? But there was a real possibility that her partner, a widower, may have assuaged his loneliness with occasional visits to a prostitute or one-night stands with acquaintances. Nice men may do these things, especially when they are lonely. I was pleased when Maxine admitted these behaviors were possible and decided to discuss condom use with her beloved. Everyone needs to be realistic in the Age of AIDS.

Lust . . .
Or A Penis Has A Head Of Its Own
(So Does The Clitoris)

I'm always amazed when gay men who have seen many friends and loved ones die, who teach and talk about AIDS and its prevention, tell me they themselves sometimes forget to practice safe sex.

Even healthcare providers who should know more about AIDS than others leave the hospital and forget to practice safe sex. They tell me that all the knowledge in the world may go right out the window in a moment of heated passion. Once they have an erection, they say, the old cliche is true — the penis has a head of its own. Knowing this, women must begin avoiding risky situations. It's only reasonable to expect that if you're alone with a man and you're flirting with each other, you're at higher risk than if you're out together with friends in a well-lit restaurant.

Trust

I treat both men and women in my practice. When we talk about AIDS and safer sex, I find that most women believe they should trust their mates. They are trustworthy themselves and can't imagine their mates might not be. It's too threatening. They want the illusion of romance and passion, the safety of shared commitment, the security of a solid relationship. Asking one's mate to use a condom may seem to shatter the illusion of fidelity.

The Desire For Pregnancy

Remaining abstinent or having sex with a condom precludes getting pregnant. For many women, the desire for pregnancy over-rides the desire to remain uninfected. I've discussed this concern in greater detail in Chapter 10, *And Baby Makes Three.*

Denial

If you are denying that your teenagers are having sex, how can they come to you and ask you for money for condoms? If a man denies his bisexuality to his wife, how can he tell her that he needs to use condoms? Even now, I still hear educated, well-read people say that AIDS is a gay man's disease, an IV drug abuser's disease, a poor person's disease. If you deny that you'll ever get infected by this virus, how can you begin to protect yourself?

Ignorance

Many people fail to understand how this disease is transmitted. Every day in my practice I hear people make statements like:

"I know the man I slept with last night was clean because he had a bath before and after sex."

"He's safe because he's a doctor."

"He's married. He wouldn't want his wife infected, would he?"

"I'm using a diaphragm."

"We only have oral sex."

In some rural areas of this country, and in Third World countries, people may have heard about AIDS, but have no idea how it's spread and certainly haven't a clue for prevention. One study in rural Uganda found that the majority of people had never used condoms, and about 15 percent had never even heard of them.

Certain cultures don't believe in the germ theory — that there are tiny little organisms which pass from one person to another. These people believe that disease is a result of the wrath of God. If you don't believe in the germ theory, how can you possibly believe in the use of condoms for the prevention of AIDS?

Ignorance about AIDS also appears among different age groups. Young people are bombarded with messages about AIDS, but people in their 60s, 70s and beyond, who may still be sexually active, may be unaware that they, too, could be at risk of infection.

A 72-year-old man I know tested positive for HIV. When questioned about how he might have been infected, it turned out that he had sex with prostitutes. None of his peers had been talking about AIDS or safer sex practices.

Poverty And Economic Dependence

Some women are worried about how to find food for their children. They can't afford a condom. In Senegal, the price of a condom is two-thirds the price of a prostitute. A half-billion condoms are supplied to the developing world every year by the United States Agency for International Development. It may sound like an enormous number, but it's not even enough to give each man age 15 to 49 one condom per year! The two million condoms donated to Uganda in 1988 were not enough for even one-third of the adult population to enjoy safer sex even once.

In wealthier educated countries, we have the luxury of thinking about how to protect ourselves. Where there is widespread poverty, just managing to live from one day to the next takes priority over preventing a disease that will kill you in 10 years' time. Why worry? You may be dead by then anyway. Millions of people are interested only in basic survival. Many have no access to health education, much less testing and treatment.

Economic dependence is not confined to underdeveloped countries. Some women who appear to be well off financially in America and other wealthy nations are totally economically dependent on their spouses. They have no training or skills with which to support themselves and may be afraid to give up a lifestyle they've become accustomed to. If they suspect their mate has been unfaithful, they may not feel they have the right to ask him to use condoms. What if his answer is to leave?

Domestic Abuse

Domestic violence and AIDS are closely intertwined, believes Surgeon General Dr. Antonia Novello. The woman who is being beaten or sexually abused by her mate is in no position to ask that man to wear a condom. Women who are victims of abuse often think they have done something to deserve it, like insulting their mate by asking him to wear a condom. If they can only figure out how not to cause their mate to get mad, like not asking him to practice safe sex, then they hope they won't get attacked.

Unfortunately abusive men can never be pleased by their partners for long. They will always find some other "reason" to beat them up. Men with deep-seated fear and hatred for women are often unfaithful. Women involved with such men run the risk of becoming infected with HIV.

These women often have low self-esteem, self-blame and a sense of helplessness. Many have drug and alcohol addictions, are often economically dependent and don't believe anyone — including themselves — can help them out of the situation.

I have a patient, Alexandra, who only comes to me in crisis. Her husband has broken her back, fractured bones in her face and has violent, prolonged and frequent sex with her. The times Alexandra has come to see me have been because of abdominal pain. I want to send her for tests, such as pelvic ultrasound, but she refuses. Although she has medical insurance, Alexandra is afraid to let her husband know that she has sought medical care. He doesn't give her any money — she has to ask and account for all money that she spends.

I'm not always able to help Alexandra with her acute medical problems because of the issues of secrecy, and I am unable to convince her to leave him. We're like actors in a deadly play. Alexandra is always in crisis and danger. And I'm helplessly standing by, worried that she's going to be murdered by her husband. How can I urge her to risk her safety by asking him whether he is monogamous, if he will consent to testing and if he will wear a condom? She obviously needs long-term counseling and a safe place to live while she learns the skills to support herself and her daughter, but she refuses to leave.

Domestic violence at every level of society is a well-kept secret, and there are few resources available to help women escape from these violent situations. We need to pay greater attention to women's issues as they relate to violence and to AIDS.

Statistics on HIV-positive women show that so far drug abusers, poor women and minority women are most susceptible to HIV infection. These are the same women who are typically found in abusive relationships. However, the FBI estimates that domestic violence touches up to 25 percent of all American families, and this abuse penetrates all economic, education and cultural levels.

"When it comes to negotiating sexuality and safer sex, we're talking about two people with equal power," says Catherine G. Lynch, Executive Director of Health Crisis Network in Miami. "Many women are in situations where they don't have that equal power, particularly if she's going to be beaten up. If she's going to get hit or lose the rent money or he's going to find another woman and she will lose her financial support, that woman isn't going to make her mate wear a condom. If she needs him for finances, for protection so someone won't break into her house, for help with disciplining the children, it's hard to negotiate for safer sex. People stay in a relationship for many reasons and sometimes are terrified to leave it; sometimes staying in that relationship is a logical choice, given the alternatives."

As a society we need to learn how to recognize, treat and prevent both the domestic violence epidemic and the HIV epidemic.

Drugs And Alcohol

We've used the term bisexual, meaning someone who has sex with both men and women. Now there's a new term — trisexual. This refers to people who are so attached or addicted to alcohol and drugs that the substance is actually a third presence in their relationship. When under its influence, they may try anything sexually. We counsel people not to have sex when they are drunk or high because they may make irresponsible choices in partners and sexual practices and don't always remember how to put on a condom properly, if at all.

Drug addicts often have sex for money, and their im-
mediate overwhelming desire for drugs obliterates their
concern for safety. Runaway teenagers often become
drug addicts. Studies show an appalling number are HIV
positive, with more female runaways testing positive than
males because they are trading sex for money, and because
women are at greater risk of acquiring this infection.

Often women may not have a drug addiction themselves, but are at risk for AIDS because they are having sex
with someone who is shooting up and using contaminated
needles.

While cocaine use does not directly cause HIV infection
from one person to another, there is a definite association.
People who are cocaine intoxicated are less inhibited in
their sexual behaviors and often forget to practice safer
sex, or have multiple partners or sell sex for drugs. All of
these practices place cocaine users at higher risk for infection and contribute to the increasing rates of heterosexual
transmission of HIV disease.

An increasingly important challenge for drug rehabili-
tation programs is how to prevent patients from acquiring
or spreading HIV. More drug abuse treatment programs
are desperately needed in this country, not only to stop
drug abuse, but also to raise the awareness level about
AIDS and help these people change their sexual behaviors.

Risk-Takers Or Russian Roulette

I once tested a man who had been married for 30 years
to a woman he said he loved dearly, and with whom he
spent almost 24 hours a day because they worked together, played together and slept together. Every now and
then their closeness drove George crazy. He would escape
for a few hours and visit a prostitute.

One day it dawned on him that not only would his wife
be distraught if she found out about his visits to these

prostitutes, but that he might, in fact, be risking her life by transmitting the AIDS virus to her.

George was almost in tears when he talked with me about his fears. He vowed he was going to stop seeing the other women. And when I tried to teach him about using condoms, he said he didn't need to know about that because he would never be unfaithful to his wife again. When George's test came back negative, he sent me a huge bouquet of flowers in gratitude for my understanding and for the good news.

A year later, George returned to my office. However hard he had tried, he couldn't stop seeing the prostitutes. He couldn't understand why he was doing it (and I think that his negative results gave him some false sense of security).

Sleeping with prostitutes gave George excitement and a feeling of beating the odds in this game of Russian Roulette. While he was beating those odds, he couldn't stop. He clearly needs counseling, but I suspect he still hasn't sought it. I'm certain that I'll see him again for testing. I can only hope that he is at least using condoms.

Some people like living on the edge. That's why they drive fast without seatbelts, take drugs, have affairs, parachute jump or eat French fries with salt when they know they're at risk for heart disease. People who crave tension and excitement in their lives may never be convinced to practice safer sex. These may be very exciting people, the kind who may attract you sexually. Think twice about how important excitement is to you.

Sex Obsession . . . Or Addiction?

"Sometimes sex becomes so over-riding for a person, so distracting that sexual energy becomes a compelling force," says Miami sexologist Lynn Leight, R.N. "I have seen clients whose drive was so forceful that they felt out of control. Their sexual need was so great that they actively sought a partner, any partner, or masturbated until there was some relief. They described the anxiety associated with their need as 'jumping out of my skin,' 'uncontrollable,' 'frightening.' "

Leight says the feelings may sound similar to those described by someone addicted to narcotics. The difference, she feels, is that substance abusers are addicted to harmful substances, but sex is inherently life-enhancing. When the need to act upon its drive becomes overwhelming, the behavior is compulsive.

I agree with Leight that sex is inherently life-enhancing, yet I know many people seem to have an overwhelming need to act out sexually or behave as if they were compelled to have sex. No matter how we describe it — sex obsession or sex addiction — sex without some form of self-control or discrimination can be harmful, as we see in case after case of AIDS.

"But Doctor, The Sex Is So Good"

"I seem to decide which relationship to stay with by how good the sex is," said Jean, a 35-year-old single mother. "I know I should have other criteria, like how good a man may be to my children, but I can't seem to get beyond the sex part."

I hear stories like Jean's frequently. Many sexually obsessive or compulsive men and women stay in or get into sexual relations that hurt them or their children — and may eventually make them ill. I ask them over and over, "Is the sex good enough to die for?"

I have an HIV-infected male patient who told me that he was a sex addict and a very religious Roman Catholic. He was a well-groomed, well-educated pharmacist who would compulsively go into adult bookstores and have anonymous sex with other men. He would feel guilty afterward and immediately go to confession. His priest, he told me, would listen to his confession, pray with him and tell him that it wasn't his fault. He was a sex addict.

I told him that what he did was illegal and that he should be put behind bars.

And then there's Sara. She was married to a lawyer who wanted to have sex several times a day. Their agreement was that she would be available to Gary at least once a day, and that he was free to find other women to meet his compulsive needs. Sara agreed to the arrangement as long as the women he chose were not known to their circle of friends and colleagues. She didn't want to be embarrassed.

I don't know if Gary used condoms or not, but I do know that both of them were at risk for contracting HIV disease, even though Sara was monogamous. Both needed counseling.

One of my teenage patients asked if I could help her with a friend, a 17-year-old girl, who had numerous sex partners. Her friend wasn't concerned about AIDS and said that she liked sex. It's apparent that this girl is having sex to fulfill needs that will never be satisfied by brief sexual encounters.

According to Ms. Leight,

> People who display sexual-compulsive behavior frequently do so for a wide variety of reasons ranging from anger to guilt, anxiety, loneliness and disenfranchisement. Often, they have a history that includes emotional or physical abuse, low self-esteem and a sense of unfulfillment. [Sometimes] they are affirming their gender, their masculinity or femininity. Generally, they are "looking for love in all the wrong places," trying to fill an unresolved void, hoping that this sexual encounter will, in some way, be magical — making them feel whole, complete and loved.

Death Wish

There are people who don't value their own lives. They don't care if they die. They may be depressed or suicidal.

They are sometimes in a relationship with an infected person, and they feel guilty because they aren't sick as well, or they feel life won't be worth living once their partner dies. A psychologist friend recently visited India where he found little interest in preventing AIDS. Some religions there accept death as going on to a more enlightened state. Believers feel that after death one will encounter a better life. Other people feel their lives have been filled with nothing but unhappiness and pain. For them, life has no value.

It's difficult to talk to people like this about safer sex without dealing with the underlying reasons for their depression and helplessness.

These are only a few of the reasons why people risk unprotected sex in spite of the dangers of the AIDS epidemic. But the bottom line for all of these reasons, I believe, is that sex gets mixed up with a lot of other emotions. We need to remember what sex is and what it is not.

As Charlotte Davis Kasl, Ph.D., says in her book, *Women, Sex and Addiction*, sex is sex, but:

Sex is not proof of being loved.

Sex is not proof of loving someone.

Sex is not proof of being attractive.

Sex doesn't make anyone important.

Sex doesn't cure problems.

Sex is not nurture.

And sex is not insurance against abandonment,
    even if you're terrific in bed.

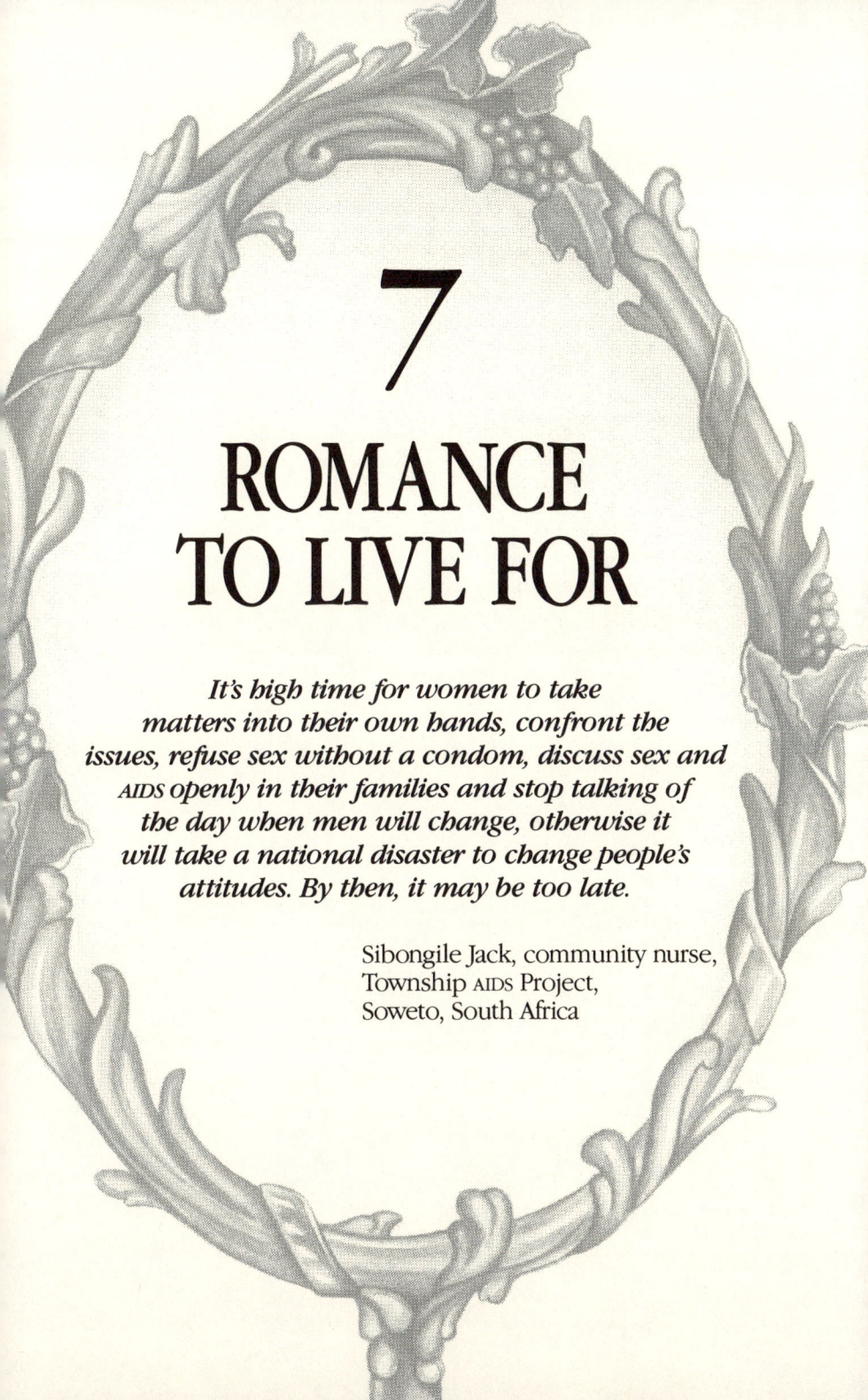

7

ROMANCE TO LIVE FOR

It's high time for women to take matters into their own hands, confront the issues, refuse sex without a condom, discuss sex and AIDS openly in their families and stop talking of the day when men will change, otherwise it will take a national disaster to change people's attitudes. By then, it may be too late.

Sibongile Jack, community nurse,
Township AIDS Project,
Soweto, South Africa

*F*rom the moment you're born, you are a sexual being. Babies like to be touched, hugged, held close, looked at, cuddled — sensations which are all expressions of love. The way we were touched as babies taught us something about our own sexuality.

As adults, we express our sexuality in many ways. Like a beautiful rainbow, our sexuality can be a colorful variety of sensual and emotional choices — with a pot of gold at the end. The pot of gold may be the moment of orgasm achieved in sexual intercourse, but this exquisite rainbow also offers an entire color spectrum of subtle delights — intimate conversation, touching, hugging, kissing, laughing and playing.

A sexual relationship can be expressed simply by the way you look at each other or touch, without ever progressing to intercourse. You can share sex that expresses love, tenderness and passion — without exchanging germ-containing fluids such as semen, vaginal secretions, urine and feces.

Sex without intercourse can be fun if you begin to use your imagination. Touching each other is a wonderful way to show affection. Think about skin as being hungry, and touching as a way to satisfy that hunger: holding hands, caressing each other, scratching each other's back, massaging the neck, head, back or feet, kissing ears, eyes, nose, even toes. You can explore each other's bodies while snuggling on the couch, reading erotic books and magazines or watching romantic videotapes.

Even with your clothes off, you can have a wonderful sexual experience without intercourse. Take a bubble bath together, sit in a Jacuzzi sipping a glass of nonalcoholic wine (so you don't get carried away), take a midnight swim in the nude. You can even fall asleep together. While it may seem hard to imagine doing any of these things without intercourse, many couples do find satisfaction in these romantic moments.

Fantasizing together is a wonderful way of expressing yourself sexually, safely. You can even do this while talking with each other over the phone.

I have a friend who was engaged to a man who lived in another city. While they saw each other as often as possible, nightly phone calls became their way of maintaining a sexual relationship. They'd often share sexual fantasies of what they would do together the next time they saw each other. The phone, for them, was a way of expressing intimacy and love. Now, even after 10 years of marriage, they find that if one of them is traveling, phone calls become their way of maintaining their love affair, long-distance.

Many older couples say that sex is better than ever, and they're not even having intercourse. They take time to explore each other's bodies, and they fall asleep touching, intertwined with each other.

The AIDS epidemic is giving us a chance to bring back old-fashioned romance. Many women tell me they would rather be touched and hugged than have intercourse. Teenagers tell me they are disappointed with intercourse. It wasn't as romantic as they thought it would be. It hurt. It left them feeling that something was missing.

Almost every day in my practice, I have to deal with the unromantic consequences of sexual intercourse, such as unwanted pregnancy, abortions, painful blisters on the vagina, drips from the penis or vagina — and AIDS.

Playing safe means that you can show love and concern for yourself and your partner. You can enjoy sex to the fullest without getting sexual diseases.

The Rest Of The Rainbow

In the 60s and 70s the sexual revolution gave "permission" to leave behind the straightlaced morals and sexual taboos of earlier generations. We broke out and went for it — directly to the rainbow's end. But the charm of the journey may have been lost en route. Sexual liaisons do not necessarily bring the intimacy and love we seek.

Before the birth control options of the sexual revolution became available, couples were obliged, out of necessity, to engage in interludes of extended foreplay. The fear of getting pregnant was so great that many dared not risk intercourse. Now we have come full circle. We can prevent pregnancy in many ways but have only celibacy and condoms to protect ourselves from AIDS.

This is a good time to define abstinence. For some people, abstinence means not being at all physical in a relationship. Even hand-holding would be considered a forbidden sexual expression.

My definition of abstinence is not having sexual intercourse. You might include kissing and some touching in your definition, or you might even include heavy petting. You need to define for yourself what you will and will not do sexually, then convey that message very clearly to your partner, preferably well before you find yourself in a passionate embrace.

The time to think about how far you'll go and what you would like from your partner is before you get into a romantic situation. It is far more important than considering the right outfit to wear, the right perfume and the right accessories. While you're putting on your jewelry, write the word "no" on the palm of your hand.

Decide in advance when you are going to say no, Lynn Leight suggests. "That will serve as a reminder in the heat of passion, when you might be tempted to throw caution to the wind, a decision you may regret in the morning. You can decide at what point of the sexual rainbow you're going to stop."

Remember, you have a basic right to set your limits. You can say no to anything you don't want to do, and no explanation is needed.

Outercourse

Perhaps you've already heard of "outercourse." It is a new word for some old-fashioned ways of expressing oneself sexually without having intercourse. You can enjoy sex filled with love, tenderness and passion that doesn't share body fluids like semen, vaginal secretions and blood.

It's important to emphasize that anal and oral intercourse **are not** outercourse.

Here are some ideas for outercourse. If you're creative you'll think of more.

- Frottage or rubbing bodies together. (Some people call this dry humping.) Some women even have orgasms while riding on their partner's thighs, elbows or feet.
- Rubbing genitals against unbroken skin. For example, some women enjoy having the penis rubbed against their breasts.
- Rubbing your own or your partner's genitals, usually to orgasm, is masturbation. This can be fun, sexy and safe.

- Sucking on the nipples of a woman who is not lactating.
- Fondling the breasts.

Women who love men with AIDS are perhaps our best teachers on how to express love without being infected.

Ellen Bukstel-Segal's husband, Doug, was among the first people with hemophilia to have been administered HIV infected blood products — before testing was available. (So was his brother. Tragically, the brothers died within six months of each other.)

When they learned that Doug was infected, the Segals were forced to make some tough decisions about their relationship. Ellen was still uninfected and had to think about herself, her three young children and about the relationship she treasured.

"Sexually, things changed dramatically," Ellen recalled. "We started using condoms, which I had never experienced before in my life. There were real concerns at that time about whether deep kissing passed on the virus so we stopped that. We talked about the sexual options that were safe for us."

As the disease began to take its toll on Doug, Ellen recalled, "We got to the point where one or the other of us would be uncomfortable. Finally, we made a decision not to have intercourse. I needed to remain well for the children. But it was very hard for Doug and me . . . in fact it was awful."

As Doug's condition deteriorated, he and Ellen engaged in new sexual intimacies such as mutual masturbation and self-gratification. Auto-eroticism became increasingly important in their relationship. "My shower massage and I got to be good friends," Ellen said.

Ellen now shares her experiences by teaching other women how significant all aspects of a sexual relationship can be. "Simply holding hands became a very important expression of our feelings," Ellen said. "When Doug held my hand, I felt that everything was okay. Most people are so caught up in their passion and arousal that they get beyond this type of intimacy. It's important to find safer ways to express their sexuality and love."

Ellen credits the precautions she and Doug took with keeping her free of ḤIV. Yet as a result of his illness, the lessons in romance they learned brought them even closer together. Doug and Ellen remained intimate until his death in 1988. By that time, "He just wasted away," Ellen said. "When we met he was six feet tall and weighed two hundred pounds; he lost more than a 100 pounds in two years."

Before his death, Doug and Ellen were dedicated to teaching others about AIDS. Ellen continues to reach out to others about AIDS. Now that she's a single woman, she is frequently asked how she protects herself. In fact, she is now involved in a long-term, mutually faithful relationship. At the start of their sexual relationship, Ellen and her partner were both tested for AIDS. Even though they both tested HIV-negative, at the beginning of their relationship they used condoms each time they made love.

"Many women like me — well-educated, middle-class — think AIDS can never happen to them," Ellen cautions. "Well, it can." She advises couples to talk about their sexual limits and expectations at the beginning of their relationship.

"Testing is a benefit, but should not be the only determining factor, since an infected person can test negative," she explained. "If I were single and uninvolved, after what I've been through, I would have no hesitation in asking my lover to use a condom. In fact, I would have nothing to do with anyone who wouldn't wear a condom."

Ellen wrote this poem to express her love for Doug:

A Precious Love

I never will forget
A time so sweet and rare

When we were so in love
With so much joy to share.

Now I feel the pain
You have each passing day
While desperately I'm wishing
For it to go away.

I look into your eyes
And feel your dark despair
Hoping that you know
How deeply that I care

Accepting the reality
Of what is meant to be
Means losing what has been
A most precious love to me.

My love, the time seems near
For us to say goodbye
And trust that our love
Will stand the test of time.

I'm feeling so alone
In a sea of desperate tears
Looking for the strength
To conquer all of my fears.

I'm angry at the thought
Of losing you this way
A part of me is dying too
As I watch you fade away.

When we try to talk
The words get in the way
I've learned that silence can reveal
The things we want to say.

My love, before you leave me
I need for you to know

I'll cling to memories never lost,
Because I love you so.

New Dating Practices

The desire to avoid HIV infection can be an opportunity to establish dating practices in which we get to know our prospective partner better before becoming sexually involved. We might be surprised by the results and attain better quality long-term relationships.

Debby, a single mother with a young daughter, devised an excellent way to protect herself when starting a new relationship.

When she met someone she was interested in, she would only make lunch dates at first to avoid a sexual situation. If after a few lunch dates she wanted to know the man better, she would consent to an evening date. Here, too, she was very careful. She would arrange for her date to pick her up at her mother's home.

"This way, men got the message early on not to expect anything more than a good-night kiss at the end of the date," Debby said. "I was in control, and if the man thought I was worth it, he'd respect my conditions. If not, I didn't really care to know him."

Debby has now become involved in a mutually faithful relationship with a man who thinks she is very special. They have had the opportunity to talk about themselves and about sex, and they have both been tested. Needless to say, Richard is now permitted to pick Debby up at her own home.

Getting Through Embarrassment

When men and women first begin to date, discussing sex and AIDS can seem awkward and embarrassing. Gail, a 35-year-old divorcee, recently began dating again. A gay man in her office had died of AIDS, so Gail knew firsthand how horrible the disease is.

Gail made a point of becoming well informed about AIDS and planned to discuss condoms and HIV testing on first dates. She had decided that a man's response would let her know right away whether there would be a second date. As she began dating, Gail found younger men were easier to talk with about safe sex than older men.

"I had a first date with a distinguished older man," Gail said. "Alan took me to a secluded oceanfront restaurant for lunch and very quickly declared his attraction for me. In my usual, straightforward fashion, I explained that in this age of AIDS I wouldn't consider a sexual relationship without getting to know the person well first and discussing condoms and testing. Well, Alan blushed to his toes, his eyes narrowed and his whole demeanor changed." Gail blushed herself while telling me the story.

Then she laughed. "Dr. Sack, he actually said he didn't know he was getting into the seamy side of life when he asked me out. He must have thought I was a prostitute or that I used drugs. There I was, as embarrassed as he was. It was awful."

Gail could not be further from the seamy side of life. Believing strongly in her cause, in the man's intelligence and in the potential for a good relationship, she persisted. She managed to break through Alan's embarrassment and convinced him of the need for honesty. After several luncheon dates they decided to pursue an intimate relationship. First, they were tested and were found to be HIV negative.

"I'm not sure where this relationship will go," Gail said, "but I feel that we have built a solid foundation of honesty and trust."

Romantic Realists

Whether Ellen, Debby, Gail and their men friends have lasting relationships or not, they have all become personal AIDS educators. I can't imagine any of them approaching sex with a partner again without frankly discussing the risks first. They are romantics who have ruled out casual sex. They want only the kind of romance they can live for.

Recently, I called a good friend, a single man who happens to be a lay minister and guidance counselor. I asked William what he would do or counsel others to do if they were dating and wanted to engage in sexual activity. He answered without hesitation: "I'd say, 'Hey, honey, I'm so attracted to you I can hardly wait to get tested. Let's go to the hospital tonight.' "

Ideally we can become so comfortable with the necessity for AIDS *testing that we can build it into the courtship process.* If we can spread information as readily as we spread the HIV virus, we may have a chance to beat this epidemic.

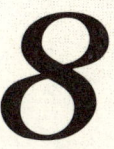

8

TESTING: THE ONLY WAY YOU'LL KNOW FOR SURE (MAYBE!)

I got the results of my HIV antibody test less than two months after I married my college sweetheart, Cookie, and less than seven weeks after she and I learned she was pregnant.

Magic Johnson, 1991

oyce is 42 years old and has been married since the age of 18 to Brad, her childhood sweetheart. They worked side by side in their family business and have a 21-year-old son. Six months ago, Brad developed shingles, a common disease, but one frequently associated with HIV. On testing for the AIDS virus, Brad was found to be positive.

In 1984 Brad had had a blood transfusion, which he claims was the cause of his infection. In the past Brad had often considered being tested for AIDS, but fear of being found positive discouraged him.

Joyce has now tested positive, too. Upon checking Brad's blood for T-cells, an indicator of how advanced the disease is, I found he had a low T-cell count. This confirmed that Brad had probably been infected years ago. Joyce's T-cell count was very high when she came to see me, signifying she was probably infected more recently.

If Joyce had known her husband was infected, she could have decided whether to practice safer sex or could have abstained. Her infection could have been prevented.

Now, since finding out that he is HIV-positive and has a limited life expectancy, Brad has left Joyce. He is angry and says he wants to taste freedom before he dies. Joyce is devastated.

She told me recently, "Brad gave me a disease I never asked for and never wanted, and now he's leaving me. How will I support myself? Where will I get health insurance? How will I take care of myself when I get ill? Who will ever want me with this disease?"

Regrettably, I have no answers to any of her questions.

Mandatory AIDS testing for everyone is not practical for many reasons. However, I encourage anyone who has any kind of concern to be tested.

A reliable test for the HIV disease wasn't developed until 1985. Before that time we could not determine if someone was infected until the individual developed symptoms of full-blown AIDS. In 1985 some public health departments began offering anonymous testing to the American population. Testing was conducted in public health offices or at alternative testing sites as health officials attempted to discover the spread of the new disease.

In 1986 the medical office I shared with another physician became one of the alternative testing sites in Miami. Anyone could be tested anonymously for a $20 fee. More than 1,000 people were tested at our office, some of whom were HIV infected, others who were at high risk but tested negative and still others who were among the worried well.

Upon entry, the patient was assigned a number and was asked to complete a questionnaire for epidemiological studies. I interviewed each person behind a closed door, offering total privacy.

We tested regulars at swingers clubs who vowed to reform and swing only with their club members if they were found negative. We tested teenagers as well as elderly men and women, some of whom were positive. Some of the women who came for testing wanted to make sure they weren't dangerous to others, to stop worrying about something they may have done in their past. Or they wanted to reassure themselves of the monogamy of their partners.

My initial question was always, "Why do you feel you need to be tested?"

And so began my education about human sexuality. I learned about married men having anonymous sex with men in parks or other places; about married and unmarried men visiting adult bookstores and having oral sex through holes in the walls; about women having love affairs with women; about gay bath houses; about men and women having extramarital affairs; about happily married men visiting prostitutes; about sexual abuse; of promiscuity beyond my wildest imagination, with some people reporting more than 1,000 partners during their lifetime.

It didn't take me long to realize that if people didn't change their sexual behavior, this little virus was going to wipe us out.

Who Should Be Tested?

Should you have an HIV test? The following Personal Risk Assessment will help you determine the answer. If you answer yes to one or more of these questions, you should seriously consider being tested.

Personal Risk Assessment

Sexual Partners

1. Have I had more than one sexual partner since 1975?

2. Have I had a sex partner who has had other sexual partners?
3. Have I had sex with anyone with AIDS or who is HIV infected?
4. Have I had sex with anyone whose past sexual behavior I do not know?
5. Have I had anal sex without using a condom?
6. Have I had vaginal sex without using a condom with someone other than a long-term, mutually faithful, uninfected partner?
7. Is my partner an alcoholic or heavy drinker? (Alcohol use and abuse lowers inhibitions.)
8. Have I ever been sexually abused or raped?

Drugs and Sex

1. Have I had sex with anyone who shoots or may have shot drugs?
2. Have I ever shared a needle to inject steroids, get tattoos or to have my ear(s) pierced?
3. Have I ever had sex after doing drugs?
4. Have I ever had sex with anyone who has had sex with anyone who shoots drugs?
5. Have I ever traded sex for drugs?
6. Have I ever shared (drug) works with anyone with AIDS or who was HIV infected?

Other Risks

1. Have I or any of my sex partners had a blood transfusion, received blood products, received an organ transplant or tried to get pregnant by artificial insemination between 1975 and 1985?
2. Do I or my sex partner handle blood, blood products or other body fluids in our jobs?
3. Have I or my partner had any sexually transmitted diseases?

4. Do I or my partner have symptoms or signs of HIV disease or a blood test that might suggest HIV disease?
5. Have I had tuberculosis (TB) or shingles (illnesses which are commonly linked with HIV-infected individuals)?

The AIDS Or HIV Test

Several kinds of tests are used to determine if a person has been infected with the HIV virus: antibody tests, antigen tests and viral cultures.

Antibody tests are the most commonly used to detect HIV. When a person is infected by the AIDS virus, the immune system produces antibodies which are found in the blood. There are two kinds of antibody tests:

- *ELISA* (Enzyme Linked Immunosorbent Assay)
- *Western Blot*

An AIDS test requires that some blood be drawn from your arm — about a teaspoonful — and that blood will be sent to the laboratory where an ELISA test will be performed.

If that ELISA is positive, meaning it detects HIV antibodies, a second ELISA will be done. If both are positive, then the Western Blot will be performed as a double check.

The ELISA test is very sensitive, picking up more than 99 percent of people who have produced antibodies to the AIDS virus. Sometimes, however, it reacts positively even when a person is uninfected. This is called a "false positive." That's why the Western Blot is performed to double check.

The Dangerous Window Period

It can take from three weeks to as long as six months for your body to produce antibodies once you've been infected with the AIDS virus. During this time, which we call the window period, you could actually be infectious, while the antibody tests falsely show that you are not infected. This is a major drawback to the antibody test.

Scientists are seeking ways to solve the problem of the window period and have developed some other tests. These, however, are at present being used only for research, or under very special circumstances. They are the p24 antigen test, the PCR or viral culture.

The p24 antigen test checks for parts of the AIDS virus itself. With the PCR, more than 100 million copies of a small amount of the virus' genetic material are made and measured. The viral culture process requires growing HIV from the blood. But the HIV doesn't always grow. Each of these tests has problems and is expensive. Therefore the ELISA and Western Blot studies will continue to be used most widely.

The antibody tests (ELISA and Western Blot) are easy to perform and are the most reliable. The cost is usually between $20 and $150 per test, depending on where you have it done. Some state public health departments perform the testing at no charge if you are unable to pay.

Your results will be reported in the following way:

- *The results are **negative.*** This can mean (1) you are virus-free and will not produce antibodies or (2) you are in the window period and need to have your blood tested again.

  We suggest that you have your blood tested six months after your last high-risk exposure (having sex without a condom or sharing a needle).

- *The results are **positive.*** This means that antibodies are present, and therefore the virus is present also. Usually there is a known risk factor. If you are entirely surprised at being infected, this may be a false positive, so please have the test repeated if you don't believe it is correct. However, these tests are usually accurate.

- *The results are* **indeterminate.** This is a grey zone in which the Western Blot test cannot be reported as being either positive or negative. This could mean that you have had a recent exposure and all of your antibodies haven't formed yet or that you are healthy and not infected.

An indeterminate finding is rare, but if that is the finding of your AIDS test, you need to have your blood retested in six weeks and again at six months. In the meantime, I suggest that you act as if you are infected to ensure that you don't infect others. That means you should not donate blood, semen, organs or have unprotected sex.

If you are told that you are HIV positive, please make sure that both an ELISA and a Western Blot test were done.

A young teenager named Vivian got chlamydia, a sexually transmitted disease, from her partner during her first sexual encounter. Her doctor wisely advised her to have an AIDS test, which she did. (By the way, minors don't need parental permission in most states for a doctor to do an AIDS test, and the results can only be given to the parent with the minor's consent.)

When the ELISA results came back, the doctor told Vivian that she had AIDS. Fortunately, he was wrong. Vivian only had a false positive ELISA. I repeated her test a few weeks later and, of course, did a Western Blot as well as the ELISA. Both were negative. Vivian was relieved, but had been traumatized emotionally by the experience. Her first sexual encounter won't be remembered as romantic and beautiful, but I hope that she's learned always to practice safer sex.

Confidential Versus Anonymous Testing

Any test or procedure performed in a doctor's office is confidential. No one, except the office workers, other healthcare workers or insurance companies should ever have access to these records.

Most insurance companies and other healthcare providers should only have access to your records with your written consent. If you have a confidential HIV test done, this is even more privileged medical information. It can be shared only if you sign a special release of information or, under very special circumstances, if a court subpoenas your records.

Some people are concerned that they may be at risk of losing important benefits if their healthcare insurance providers and/or their employer find out they had an HIV test. These individuals prefer not to have an HIV test on their record, regardless of whether the test was positive or negative.

If you are concerned about confidentiality, you can have the test performed anonymously. This means you are never asked your name, address or social security number. For example, in public health departments, you are assigned an identifying number. When you return for your results, you ask for the results for your number, rather than your name.

Private doctors' offices usually cannot give you a number since most labs that run the tests will not accept a number into their computer recordkeeping systems.

However, because I believe strongly in testing, I offer my patients a way to do it anonymously. If it is easier for them, they merely make up a name, and that name cannot be traced back to their medical record. I sometimes recommend they use their first name and their mother's maiden name, so they are less apt to forget it. Other doctors have alternative ways of doing this.

These are simple, practical ways of having the test performed anonymously.

Informed Consent

Many states have a legal requirement that a person can be tested for AIDS only after giving informed consent.

This means counseling must precede the test. At the time of testing, a healthcare provider is required to talk with the individual about the reasons for having the test, to explain what the test means and to counsel the individual about prevention of the disease.

Some states require that test results must be given face-to-face. In many states, it's illegal to get the test results over the telephone, although I know it is sometimes done. The psychological impact of finding out that one has an HIV-positive test could be devastating, and the results should be shared in the presence of a trained counselor or physician.

Healthcare workers also use the office visit as an opportunity to talk about prevention if the individual tested negative; to discuss the procedure for a follow-up test if needed; or what steps to take if the individual tested positive.

The only people who do not need to give informed consent are: donors of blood, semen or tissues; or people entering the military. The court can also order a test to be performed without consent — for example, on someone accused of rape.

Don't make the mistake of thinking that if you visit your doctor and receive a physical exam with blood tests, you will automatically be tested for HIV. You will not, unless you have been counseled and given your consent to have the test done. You'll know if you've been tested by a doctor for HIV.

At this time insurance companies can test you without consulting you or even letting you know you are being tested. They will not give you your results, but they will send them to your physician if you ask them to. Some people think if the insurance company takes blood from them and then issues a life or health insurance policy, they must be HIV free. Don't count on it. Because they do not test everyone who applies for insurance, some HIV positive people will be insured.

If you learn you are HIV infected, you may not know when you got the AIDS virus, who gave it to you, whether you will get AIDS, how sick you are or how long you will live. The test only informs you that you have been infected with the virus and that you can pass this virus on to someone else. You will not be able to donate blood, organs or semen.

If you test positive, you should find a doctor who is knowledgeable about HIV disease. You'll need a complete physical examination and some blood tests to determine where you are in the spectrum of HIV disease so that you can get the best possible healthcare. Remember, AIDS has now become a chronic, manageable disease, and we can now prevent many of the opportunistic infections that people died from previously.

If you test negative now, it doesn't mean you will always remain negative. If you are practicing unsafe sex with an infected partner, or if you share IV needles with an infected person, you can still become infected in the future.

Before being tested, consider the following:

- How much will the test cost? Will I need to pay for it in cash? (This is often the case at anonymous test sites.)
- Will the test be done confidentially or anonymously?
- Who will know the results?
- How will the results be reported?
- If I test positive, who would I have to share this knowledge with?
- Can I expect psychological support from my friends or family, or should I see a professional?
- Where will I go for my healthcare?
- If I'm pregnant, what are my feelings about maintaining the pregnancy or my beliefs about abortion?

Notifying Partners

It seems reasonable to expect that a responsible person who learns that she or he is HIV infected would tell past, current and future partners, but it's not always that easy. Many people feel ashamed about having this disease, guilty that they may have passed it on to another partner or angry that the partner may have given it to them. They may be denying that they have the disease. Sometimes telling a partner about the infection means confessing a side of life of which the partner was unaware.

How do you tell a past or current partner that you are HIV infected? Telling a sexual partner that you are HIV infected and may have infected him is very difficult. To make matters worse, you might not know how to find past sexual partners.

I asked one of my infected female patients where she might have got the infection. She thought it might have been one of two sexual partners, both of whom had moved. One of them had infected her, and one of them may have been infected by her. She had no way of tracing them. If they are still sexually active and do not know they are infected, they could be infecting many women.

My patient, Jonathan, was hospitalized for pneumonia. While there, he agreed to be tested for HIV. He tested positive. When I talked with him about the need to tell his wife, he was at a loss at how to start. He had so much to say: that he was infected, that he was a bisexual having an affair with a man, that he was going to die and that he may have given his wife this disease.

That was a great deal to tell someone you'd been married to for more than 10 years. Understandably, Jonathan avoided telling Laura for several weeks despite my continual urging. I was concerned that he would infect her, if he hadn't already. Finally when I threatened to send a certified letter to Laura telling her husband's HIV status, he agreed to bring her to talk with me.

I would not have minded if Jonathan avoided telling Laura that he was bisexual. That was his private issue, and he could make up any story he liked as far as I was concerned. My concern as a doctor was to protect his wife from possible infection through unsafe sex.

Fortunately Laura tested negative.

If Jonathan hadn't told his wife, I would have told her. As a doctor, I feel that I have a responsibility to protect human life, even if it means breaching patient confidentiality. In Florida and at least 12 other states, the law protects doctors in these situations. We aren't required by law to notify partners, but if we do, we can't be sued for breach of confidentiality. As of 1990, only two states have imposed on physicians a legal duty to warn spouses that they are at risk for HIV infection from their partner. (If you want to know the laws in your state, call the HIV division of your state health department or the state medical society.)

For those people who find it too difficult to tell another person, public health departments in some states may be able to help. Individuals may be retested to verify the results and if the results are positive, the health department will ask for the names and addresses of any past sexual or needle-sharing partner who may have been infected.

Then a health department representative will personally visit each person, explaining that he or she may have been exposed to HIV through a past relationship. This is done with complete confidentiality. Each person contacted will be counseled and offered HIV testing. Even though mandatory notification programs are under discussion, current partner notification programs are voluntary. But such programs are only effective if the infected person is willing to share information about past relationships.

The Wrong Message

I'm concerned that the issue of HIV testing is somehow being mixed up with feelings of shame and guilt. I have patients who are afraid that they'll be recognized if they go for testing. They don't want their personal doctors to know and they surely don't want their friends or co-workers to know. That's why I and others have tried to set up a system that assures their anonymity.

I don't have to know who a person is or what they do for a living if they come to me for testing. I just need to help them understand what they've done to cause their fear of having been infected and show them how, if they test negative, they can prevent ever becoming infected. If they test positive, at least we can begin to work together to assure as long and healthy a life as possible, without passing the disease on to others.

I know a nurse who lives in a small western community. Betty is single and recently had unprotected sex with a younger man during what she described as a "wonderfully passionate evening." She's also had several incidents at the hospital where she works of being stuck by a needle used on a patient. Yet Betty is so afraid of being tested for HIV, she'd prefer to live in fear rather than discover the truth. She's concerned that in her close-knit town, someone will find out she's been tested.

I've suggested that she send her blood to me in Miami, or that she go to the health department or doctor in another town, where she'll be less likely to see someone she knows. There are many ways of being tested if you really want to be.

Recently a patient came to see me about a cold she couldn't seem to shake. Her nagging cold and cough worried her, particularly since she had had a blood transfusion in 1985 before national screening of the blood supply for HIV. Jessica was terrified that she might have AIDS. She told

me she had previously asked her gynecologist if he would
test her for HIV, because she had had this blood transfusion. He had told her, "Don't be silly, you don't have AIDS.
And even if you are positive, there's nothing you can do,
so why know?"

Jessica's fears were not allayed by this doctor's dismis-
sive comments. She had been obsessing for months, inter-
preting every symptom as AIDS related. I tested her and
she tested negative.

Fortunately Jessica's doctor was correct about her not
being infected, but his answer to her was wrong on both
counts. First, she wasn't being silly. Second, there are
things you can do if you are positive.

In Jessica's case, the test results affected her decision
about having more children. It also affected her relationship with her husband. If she tested positive for HIV, she
could take steps to protect her husband. And she could
begin to take medications available to help prolong her life.

I believe Jessica's gynecologist was wrong. If you want a
test and your doctor doesn't want to test you, convince
him or her that you need the test or find another healthcare source.

*Anyone who has the slightest concern about carrying the AIDS
virus should be tested. It's the only way we can stop this epidemic.*

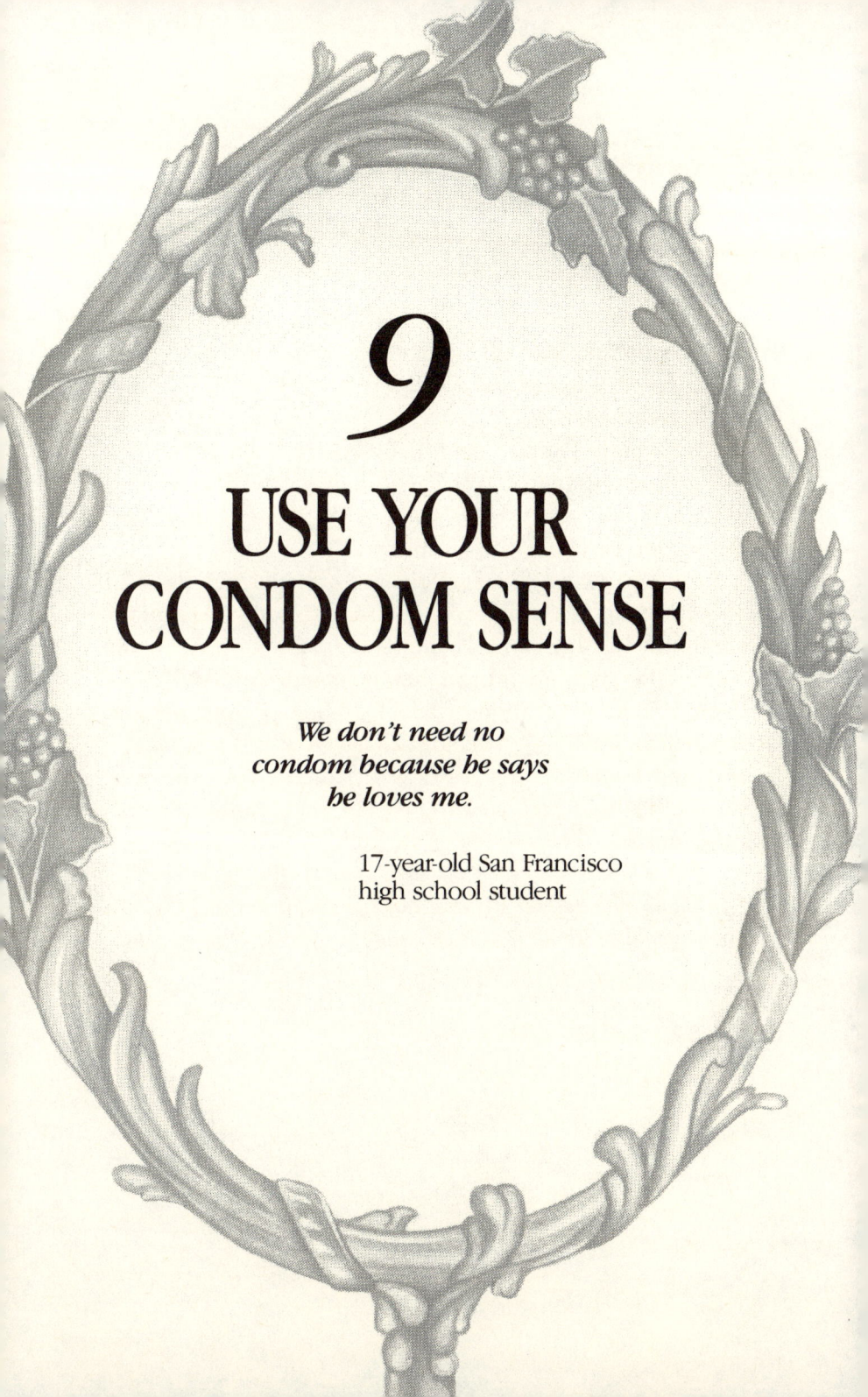

9

USE YOUR CONDOM SENSE

*We don't need no
condom because he says
he loves me.*

17-year-old San Francisco
high school student

*M*aggie is 26, vivacious, HIV infected, single and lonely. Yet she manages to stay in a good mood in spite of her condition. My staff and I can't help liking her and feeling sad that the disease is ravaging her body in spite of the fact that her behavior is completely irresponsible.

Maggie was one of the first people to alert us that we needed to educate everyone about condoms. She told us that she frequently goes to bars and that men always try to pick her up. When she asks them about having sex with condoms, they laugh and say they don't need to worry.

We thought she ought to be out in public wearing a sign saying, "Look at me! I'm healthy looking, full of fun, sexy and HIV positive." She'd stop people in their tracks of denial.

When she came into our office a few months ago, she was pregnant and needed to take a long, hard look at whether or not to terminate her pregnancy.

It was an agonizing decision for her. She had always expected that her life would include marriage and a child. Now she was pregnant and HIV positive. At first she wanted to keep the baby, but eventually decided to have an abortion, because she was single, would soon get ill and would have no support. She didn't really know the father very well. She told us the condom had broken and she hadn't told him about the pregnancy because his reaction to her keeping or aborting the fetus wasn't a factor in her decision. She expected nothing from him. She cried a lot and we cried with her.

Recently, I learned more about Maggie from one of her friends. Her life story included sexual abuse as a child, and many subsequent sexual problems as she entered her teens. She had been very promiscuous until she began living with a bisexual man a few years ago. When he became ill, Maggie was tested and found to be HIV infected. Her lover has since died of AIDS.

Maggie remained sexually active and soon began having an affair with a married man. She'd been in this relationship for at least a year before telling Matt she was HIV infected. Besides Matt, Maggie has another boyfriend who knows she's HIV positive and has had several other casual affairs. She rarely tells her partners of her HIV status and doesn't always use a condom. The father of her child had no idea of her HIV status.

Recently Maggie was diagnosed as having cervical cancer, common in HIV-infected women. She refused to have a hysterectomy to remove the cancer. She still clings to the dream of marrying and having a child.

How many people have been exposed to AIDS because of Maggie? Her married lover, his wife and their children; her sexual partners and their sexual partners — we will never know the rest of this sad, chilling story. One of my colleagues thinks of her as "the serial killer."

Condoms . . . Or Thanks To Casanova

When I grew up in South Africa, "FLs" or French Letters, as condoms were called, were never discussed. In fact, when one would go to buy an FL, all you had to do was flip a quarter, place it on the counter and the drugstore clerk knew exactly what you wanted. In our culture we never spoke about sex. We used condoms, but didn't talk about them.

My friends tell me things weren't so very different in America. With the advent of the pill and IUD, condoms lost their popularity as a means of birth control.

But with the AIDS epidemic, things have changed. In fact more than 418 million condoms were sold in the United States in 1991. And whether you're on the pill, use an IUD or other form of birth control, you still need to use a condom to protect against infection from HIV and other sexually transmitted diseases.

What Are Condoms?

Condoms — sometimes called rubbers, prophylactics, sheaths or French Letters — are protective barriers that cover the penis. They have been used for centuries to prevent pregnancy and infection. As early as 1350 B.C., condoms were used as a decoration and occasionally were used to produce penile or vaginal stimulation.

In the 16th century Gabriel Fallopius designed medicated linen sheets for the tip of the penis for the purpose of preventing venereal diseases. By the 17th century condoms were used for contraception as well. They were made of animal gut, hemmed at one end, and were wryly referred to as ". . . an armor against love, but a gossamer against infection."

Casanova, who lived between 1725 and 1798, was among the first to popularize condoms for contraceptive use. In the 1840s condoms were made of rubber; since the 1930s, they have been made out of latex. The first condoms were washable, so they could be reused, but now they're disposable and should never be reused.

Today condoms come in many different shapes, sizes, types, colors and flavors. There are even female condoms available. Natural skin condoms are not effective in preventing the spread of viruses — they are too porous, and tiny viruses can leak through them.

While the scientific community searches for cures for AIDS and other sexually transmitted diseases like herpes, we must protect ourselves and others from being infected. Prevention is our only armor. The proper use of condoms with each act of sexual intercourse can reduce but cannot eliminate the risk of sexually transmitted diseases.

For the male, the condom reduces the risk of the penis becoming infected from contagious cervical, vaginal, vulval or rectal secretions. For the receptive partner (female or male), the condom prevents the semen from coming into direct contact with the vagina, mouth or rectum. The condom also covers any open sores on the head or shaft of the penis and contains urethral discharge.

Buying Condoms

We've come a long way from the days when you'd sneak into a drugstore to buy condoms. Now condom boutiques are popping up all over.

When a condom boutique opened in Coconut Grove, a neighborhood in Miami, I took a friend of mine to see it. Irene has been married for 20 years and has used condoms all those years to prevent pregnancy. But she'd never bought a condom herself. It was always her husband's responsibility.

Irene thought she'd be embarrassed to come with me to a condom store but curiosity got the best of her. Within 10 minutes, she felt comfortable enough to ask the store clerk about the differences between ribbed and non-ribbed, the variety of flavors they stocked and the range of prices. She happily walked out with a sackful of new and different condoms, saying how much fun it would be to shop there with her husband. Irene hopes her daughter learns to feel as comfortable about buying a condom as she did.

If you don't have a condom boutique in your area, you and your friends might go to several drugstores and buy a variety of them. Get together to compare prices, types and maybe even sizes! Buying condoms needn't be shameful or embarrassing if you remember it's about saving your life. After the first few times your embarrassment will fade. Even if it doesn't, it should be easy to choose between a moment of blushing and a lifetime of disease.

It doesn't matter how old you are or what sex you are — anyone can buy a condom. They are available at drugstores, some grocery stores, gas stations, convenience stores and usually hotel gift shops. Look for them at vending machines in ladies' rooms. There are even mail order condom companies advertised in some magazines, should you prefer to "shop at home."

When buying a condom, make sure the package states that it can be used for prevention of disease and pregnancy. Some condoms are intended just to enhance sexual pleasure and are not a good barrier for pregnancy and prevention of disease. Some are sold as gag gifts. Don't trust them to be effective in preventing infection.

Look at the date on the condom package. There should be either a manufacturer's date or an expiration date. Do not use a condom after the expiration date, or more than two years after the manufacturer's date.

Once you've bought the condoms, they must be stored in a cool dry place since they do deteriorate, just like a balloon. Extremes of temperature will make the latex brittle or gummy. Do not store condoms in your purse, wallet or glove compartment of your car. Don't use a condom if it's brittle, yellow or looks damaged in any way.

There are now some pretty, feminine condom holders on the market for women to keep in their purses. They resemble a compact, so no one needs to know what's inside. You can even buy condom jewelry, such as necklaces and earrings that look like costume jewelry but have a condom hidden in the back; or a key ring that holds keys and a condom.

Who Should Use A Condom?

If you want to prevent pregnancy, a condom is one of several birth control options. If you want to minimize your risk of being infected by a sexual partner, the condom may be your best option. Keep in mind that infertile or sterilized women are five times less likely than unsterilized women to use condoms and therefore they face a greater risk of contracting AIDS and other sexually transmitted diseases.

Who *Doesn't* Need To Use A Condom?

You don't need to use a condom if you're not having intercourse. You also don't need to use a condom if you fulfill all of the following criteria:

- You are in a mutually monogamous relationship. That is, neither you nor your partner is having sex with anyone else.
- Neither of you has had sex with anybody else for six months or longer.
- You've both been tested and are both HIV negative.
- You intend to remain in your monogamous relationship.
- You trust that your partner will remain faithful as well.
- Neither of you is injection drug abusers.
- Neither of you has had a recent blood transfusion or accidental blood exposure.

Everybody else should wear a condom, whether they are having vaginal, anal or oral sex.

With all these strict criteria, you may be saying to yourself that it seems almost everyone should be wearing a condom. You're right. But think about it. Even though your sexual partner looks and feels healthy, he or she could still be carrying the virus and you need to use a condom to protect yourself from being infected.

Warning: Condoms Are Not 100 Percent Safe

Condoms are not 100 percent safe, either because they're not manufactured properly or because they're not used correctly.

Manufacturer's Failure

The United States Food and Drug Administration (FDA) tests condoms. The agency has forced condom manufacturers with an unacceptable number of failures to withdraw their products from the market. In 1987 the FDA undertook an expanded program to inspect latex condom manufacturers, repackagers and importers to evaluate their quality control and testing procedures.

At present the FDA checks condoms randomly. They test a batch of 1,000 at a time, and if no more than four of them are found to be defective, that manufacturer's condoms are considered safe. The average failure rate of condoms that have met the FDA approval is 2.3 per 1,000. The same standards apply for condoms made in other countries. If the FDA finds that two or more batches of condoms from a foreign company are defective, that company is banned from bringing any other shipments into the country.

Because 2.3 condoms out of 1,000 may have leaks, condoms are not considered foolproof for preventing pregnancy; nor are they foolproof for stopping infection.

Condoms are tested randomly by the manufacturer as well as the FDA. The condom is filled with water. Naturally, if it leaks, it is defective. You should *not* try this test yourself on a condom you plan to use, because you may damage it in the process.

User Failure

User failure is caused by *not* using a condom for each act of sexual intercourse.

My patients often say they use condoms. But when asked if they use condoms 100 percent of the time, they usually say, "Yes, except when I'm too drunk or high . . . except when sex got too hot and we forgot . . . except when I was with this man who washes before and after sex . . . except when I didn't feel like it."

It's during those "except" times that women can get pregnant, get syphilis, herpes, gonorrhea or AIDS. Remember, a one-time lapse in condom use can have lethal implications.

The second major reason for user failure is that the condom is not put on at the correct time. The condom must be placed on the penis as soon as the man has an erection and before any genital contact is made. It is not good enough to put it on just before ejaculation, because the virus is found in the pre-ejaculate fluid as well. This is the small amount of fluid, sometimes called the pre-cum, which is released from the man's penis even before he has ejaculated.

The third reason for user failure is that the condom is used incorrectly. Here is what you need to know about using a condom correctly:

1. Use a condom from start to finish of lovemaking.
2. Open the package carefully. Don't use your teeth, scissors or sharp nails. Don't tear the condom.
3. The condom should be placed on the penis as soon as it is erect and before it is inserted into the mouth, vagina or anus. Do not place a condom on a soft penis or the condom will slip off.

4. If the man is uncircumcised, pull back the foreskin before putting on the condom.

5. The condom needs a half-inch at the end of it to contain the semen. Some condoms have a reservoir for this purpose. If the condom doesn't, keep a half-inch between the tip of the penis and the end of the condom. Squeeze out any air (from the condom, not the penis).

6. When placing the condom, roll it to the base of the penis. Use a condom that covers the whole of the penis. Some condoms, called "stubbies," are designed specially for oral sex and are not intended for vaginal or anal sex.

7. Always use a spermicide *with* a condom, not in place of the condom. (Spermicides with nonoxynol-9 are thought to add extra protection against HIV infection.)

8. Some condoms are lubricated, either with silicone, spermicidal jelly or cream. But if you need more lubrication, do not use oil-based lubricants such as petroleum jelly, cooking oil, vegetable oil, mineral oil, massage oil, butter or cream. These will damage the condom. Also because the virus is sometimes found in saliva, it is prudent not to use saliva for lubrication.

   Instead, use water-soluble lubricants such as KY jelly or HR jelly. Your local drugstore pharmacist can help you find a water-soluble lubricant.

9. After sex, make sure the condom remains on the penis until the penis is withdrawn. The penis should be withdrawn slowly directly after ejaculation. Then you or your partner can remove the condom by rolling it off, away from your body. Wash hands and penis after taking off the condom, so the semen won't spill on you. Do not fall asleep with the penis inside you. While it may be romantic, it can be deadly

if the condom slips off inside the vagina, spilling infected semen.

10. Look at the condom before discarding it to make sure it hasn't broken. If it has torn, or if it should slip off during intercourse, do not douche because the virus will be spread up into the cervix. Place an extra amount of spermicidal jelly (with nonoxynol-9) or foam into your vagina or anus.

11. Wrap up the condom and discard it where others will not have to handle it. Don't flush it down a toilet, because it can block the sewer.

12. Don't reuse condoms. If you're going to have sex again, use a clean condom.

Please note that if you engage in oral sex, you should use a condom on the penis, but do not use one with nonoxynol-9. Research has not yet been concluded on the effects of this spermicidal jelly on the human body if it is ingested. Many people who use the spermicidally lubricated condoms for oral sex report some oral irritation, including a burning or numbing sensation, nausea or cramps. Rectal irritation has also been reported by both women and men.

Nonoxynol-9 is known to produce vaginal and rectal irritation and inflammation, and this in turn can increase the chance of HIV transmission. If you have experienced any of these symptoms after using nonoxynol-9, discontinue using it. An alternative is to ask your partner to put the nonoxynol-9 inside the condom.

Condoms For Men And Women

To make condoms inviting, manufacturers have come up with a wide range of condom choices. They may be lubricated or nonlubricated, flavored or nonflavored, colored, ribbed or smooth, tapered or nontapered. Some even glow in the dark. Some have reservoirs on the end and some have spermicidal jellies or are prelubricated.

In the past women had to rely on men wearing condoms. But now condoms are being made especially for women to wear. The female condom is expected to protect against pregnancy and is also the first device made for women to protect against AIDS and other diseases.

We should welcome female condoms and the power they give us to prevent HIV transmission. No longer will women need to rely on the male's willingness to use a condom. True, some people believe that men should bear a greater responsibility for protecting against disease and pregnancy. However, if we women can protect ourselves, let's do it. A friend of mine always asks to sit near the exit door on an airplane. Why? Because she prefers to trust herself to react quickly in times of crisis, rather than depending on someone else to be responsible for her life. In the same way, we can come to rely upon ourselves in preventing AIDS in women.

Basically, there are three types of female condoms awaiting FDA approval. Two are designed to be inserted into the vagina prior to sex, and the third is anchored by a bikini panty, and is inserted into the vagina either prior to sex or by the thrusting penis.

One of the new condoms is called The Reality, which I think is a splendid name. Wearing a condom may not be romantic to some, but the reality is that a condom is needed for our continued survival.

The Reality, which is already in use in Switzerland, is a pouch that lines the vagina and is anchored inside and outside the body by two flexible rings at either end. The pouch is made from transparent polyurethane and is seven inches long and lubricated. The rubber ring at the closed tip is flexible so that it may be inserted into the vagina, up against the cervix, much like a tampon or diaphragm is inserted. The ring at the open end of the sheath remains outside of the body, and holds the condom in place.

Another new vaginal pouch on the horizon is called Woman's Choice. This is similar to The Reality except it's made from latex, and there is a thickened rubber tip at the closed end instead of the flexible ring. This is inserted into the vagina with a special applicator, much like a tampon.

The Bikini Condom is a panty that covers the genital area and has a built-in pouch which is inserted into the vagina before intercourse. The pouch can be inserted by the woman prior to intercourse, or by the male thrusting his penis into the vagina. This condom garment is actually a unisex device, since it may be worn by the male or female, becoming either a vaginal liner or penis cover.

The polyurethane protects both the man and the woman. It prevents semen from contacting the woman's labia, vagina or cervix, protecting her from pregnancy and sexually transmitted diseases. And because the man's penis doesn't touch the woman's vagina, it also protects the man.

Who should use the female condom?

If you are sexually active and want birth control and protection against disease, if you are allergic to latex condoms or if you would like to take the responsibility for protecting yourself and others, then you should learn about the female condom.

The Down Side
Of Female Condoms

No one I know has used female condoms yet because they were not approved by the FDA at the time this book was published. But based on what I've read, there may be some women who won't try the female condom.

I've met many patients who don't like to use tampons, diaphragms or contraceptive sponges. They are uncomfortable inserting anything into the vagina. They also may be embarrassed by having a ring hang outside of the vagina, because it looks "weird." I've also learned that the condom may make a slight squeaky noise.

The biggest disadvantage, as far as I am concerned, is its expected cost, about $2.25, or about three times the price of a male condom. This may place the female condom out of reach of the woman who needs it the most: the indigent woman who cannot afford to buy one. If you use two female condoms a week, the price will be about the same as birth control pills.

The Up Side
Of Female Condoms

I believe the advantages of female condoms will far outweigh the disadvantages. First, the female condom does not require fitting by a healthcare professional, as the diaphragm does, and it doesn't require precise placement over the cervix. Besides allowing women more control over what happens to their bodies, the female condom offers these advantages:

- Polyurethane is stronger than the latex used in male condoms, and it is softer, thinner and odor free. Research to date shows that because it is stronger and less porous, there is less chance of the female condom breaking or the semen or virus leaking through into the vagina.
- Resistance to oils, allowing use of any lubricant, including baby oil and vaseline as well as water-based products, such as KY jelly, and the vaginal estrogen creams some women require after menopause.
- Greater protection from sexually transmitted diseases, such as herpes, because it covers the labia and the urethra.
- For birth control purposes, it can be removed immediately — unlike the diaphragm or sponge — but it can be inserted ahead of time. Also it does not require a male erection for its insertion.
- Because it is thinner than the male latex condom, it feels more natural to both partners.

- If the female condom slips off, it still covers the penis, continuing to prevent contact between the penis and the vagina.

Once approved by the FDA, it is expected that female condoms will be very popular. Twenty-five percent of the 418 million condoms sold in America last year were bought by women. It is estimated that female condoms will be regularly used by two to three million women.

If you plan to purchase the condom when it becomes available, please *practice* before actually using it during a sexual encounter.

It's important to remember that you should never reuse a condom, no matter what type you choose to use.

I Don't Play Russian Roulette

I hope that everyone who reads this book will make a promise to herself that there is no negotiating for condom use. Either your partner uses a condom or you don't have sex. If a woman doesn't look out for herself, who will? We must learn how to say no to a partner who won't use condoms. It's either that or abstinence.

A woman I know, who is in her late 40s, brought up the subject of condom use during an elegant dinner date with a somewhat older, well-educated and polished corporate executive. At the word condom, he turned bright red, and said, "Just how many men have you slept with?" For a moment, she was stunned by his response, as if in his eyes she had suddenly been degraded. Seeing there was no way to break through his negative attitude toward condom use, she decided not to see this man again.

Of course, it may be embarrassing to ask a man to use a condom, especially if you do not know him well. But the man you don't know really well is exactly whom you need to ask to use the condom. Embarrassment won't kill you, but unsafe sex will.

I've counseled many men and women who have never used a condom, and suddenly find themselves on the dating scene after a divorce or death of a spouse. Teenagers also have come to me for instruction. Many people are embarrassed to talk about the subject, but the problem is that some men don't know how to wear a condom and some women are afraid to ask them to.

If you've never used a condom, buy one and practice with it before having sex. Men can practice on themselves; women on a dildo, banana or cucumber.

Please don't have sex when drunk or high since you may not use the condom, or you may not use it correctly.

Be Prepared

Let's talk about some of the objections you may hear from your partner about using condoms. If you know beforehand what some objections may be, you can prepare your answer. Just remember: you don't have to have sex without a condom.

Ron is a handsome single man and you are wildly attracted to him. In the heat of passion, Ron says, "Honey, are you on the pill?"

You reply, "Yes, I'm on the pill (or diaphragm or IUD). But, Ron, once I saw a poster of a woman saying *'I have AIDS and all I was worried about was pregnancy.'* Ron, let's use a condom in addition to my birth control method, so that both of us can be protected from getting infections as well as prevent having an unwanted child."

You have a condom and offer to put it on him.

He says, "I don't use condoms."

You can say, "Well then, we'll have to think of other things to do because I never make love without a condom."

Maybe Ron will come back in a week after having thought over what you said. This time he'll come with a condom because he would like to have a serious relationship with you and he realizes you weren't only protecting your-self, you were protecting him as well.

Then there's Jeff. After a romantic, candlelight dinner, you realize that all signs are green for a wild evening in bed. But before you leave the restaurant, you tell him that you don't make love without a condom. Jeff, who just recently was divorced and has seldom had to use condoms, says, "I don't have a condom with me."

You answer, "Then let's go and buy some."

He says, "It's too embarrassing to buy condoms."

You say, "I know it's embarrassing, so I'll come with you. You paid for the dinner. I'll pay for the condoms."

He says, "I don't really like using condoms."

You say, "There's all different kinds. Let's try a few of them and find one you like."

Jeff agrees to try out a variety of condoms, and your relationship is off to a good start.

Philippe is a romanticist. When you raise the question of using a condom, he says, "I love you, and I would never hurt you."

You say, "I love you, too, and I know you wouldn't know-ingly hurt me, but some people have diseases they don't know about. I won't make love without a condom."

He says, "It's not romantic to put it on and it interrupts foreplay, and I can't keep an erection when I put on a condom."

You say, "Let me put it on, darling, as a part of foreplay," or "I don't feel romantic when I'm scared about getting pregnant or getting AIDS or sexually transmitted diseases."

Together you learn that sharing the experience of put-ting on a condom can be erotic.

Poor Irwin. When you tell him you won't have sex without a condom, he says, "But I'm allergic to them, and they make my penis itchy and swollen."

Having rehearsed for every possible answer, you're ready for that excuse. You say, "I read that you can 'double-bag.' That means if you are allergic to the latex brands, you can first put on a natural skin condom and then put the latex on top. That way the latex won't touch your skin and you won't have a painful reaction."

He says he doesn't know if he's allergic to latex, or to the spermicidal jelly. You can test that by putting a small amount of spermicidal jelly on his lip. If he's allergic, his lip will swell, and you'll know not to use condoms with spermicidal jelly inside of them. You can still use the jelly outside of the condom. (By the way, if you are allergic to latex condoms, you can reverse the double bagging, and have your partner put the latex on first, followed by the natural skin condom. If it's the spermicidal agent you are allergic to, have him put it inside his condom.)

You're reading this book and now realize that you should have been using condoms in your long-term relationship with Larry. When you tell him that you want to begin using them, he says, "But we are true to each other."

You say, "I know, but we've both had sex partners in the past. And when we sleep with each other, we're really sleeping with each other's previous sex partners, too. I think we could enjoy each other more if we didn't have to worry and I've decided that, from now on, I won't have sex without a condom." You can promise him that once you've been together for six months, you can both be tested for HIV, and if you test negative, and are still true to each other and aren't using IV drugs, then you can throw away the condoms.

He says, "But, sweetheart, sex isn't as much fun with a condom — it's like wearing a raincoat in the shower."

You say, "There are some condoms available now that might enhance your sensitivity, especially the lubricated ones. But even if they do reduce your sensitivity, just remember, you can't feel anything when you're dead." You can also tell him that some people find condoms help reduce pre-ejaculation, and that the rim of the condom may help some men maintain an erection longer.

Bruno shows his true colors when you bring up the subject of condoms. He says, "You can see that I'm not one of those guys. I don't have AIDS and I'm insulted that you would even think that. Are you implying that I have a disease? I never wear condoms." (Warning: This is the man you should worry about the most. If he won't wear a condom with you, he hasn't worn a condom with any other partner. And you are trusting your life to someone who doesn't want to make love to you, he just wants to screw you.)

You say, "Well, I guess we're not going to bed tonight because I never have sex without a condom." Bruno is clearly not worth dying for.

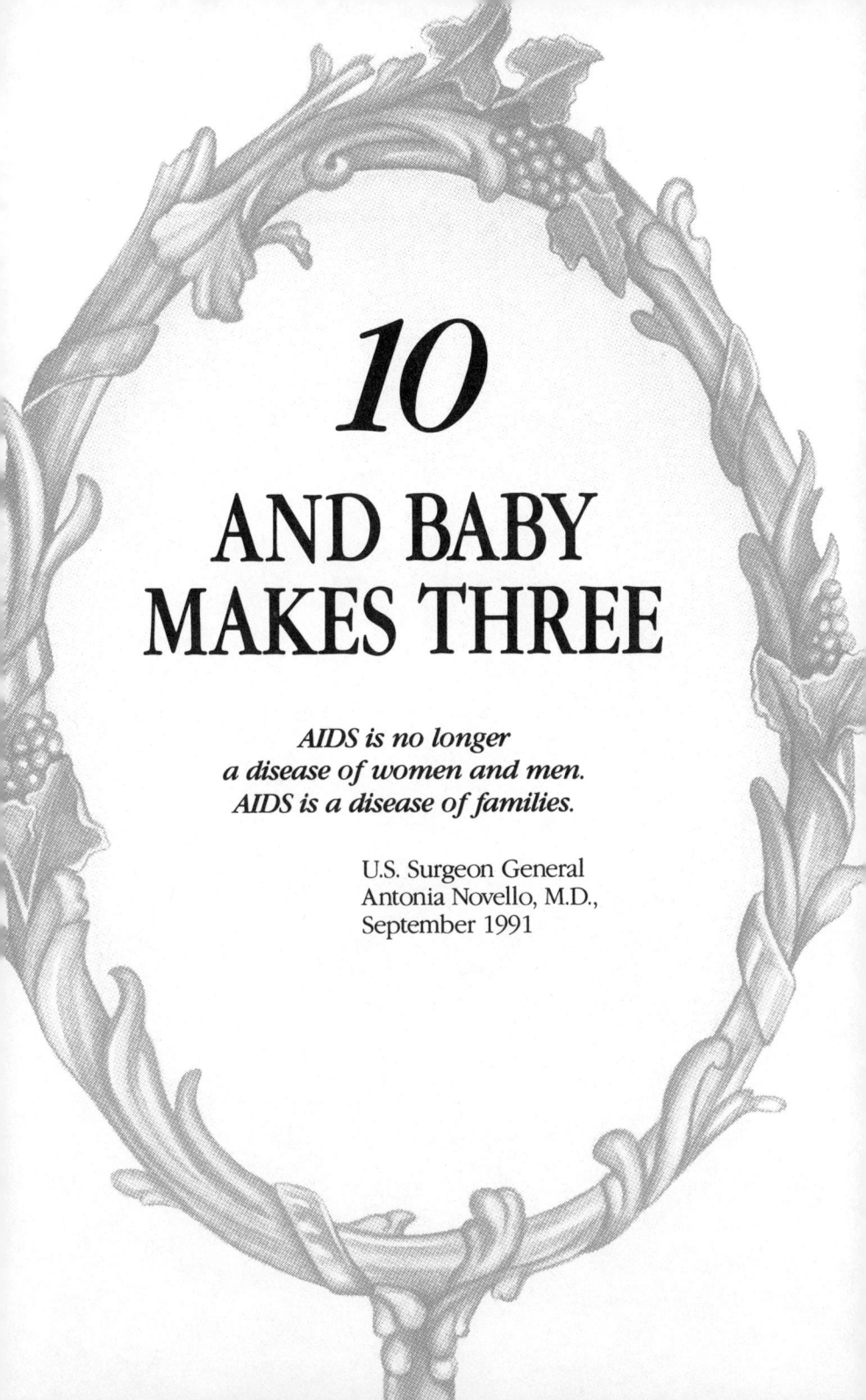

10

AND BABY
MAKES THREE

*AIDS is no longer
a disease of women and men.
AIDS is a disease of families.*

U.S. Surgeon General
Antonia Novello, M.D.,
September 1991

*H*aving a baby isn't as simple as it used to be. Since the AIDS epidemic began, an increasing number of women are beginning to realize that the topic of HIV should enter into any discussion about getting pregnant. In fact, the vast majority of women with AIDS are of childbearing age — AIDS is the number five killer of women in this age group. This means that several thousand HIV-infected women will become pregnant each year, and the number worldwide is increasing dramatically. Some won't find out about their disease until they are pregnant and tested for the virus.

Consider Martha, a 20-year-old mother-to-be, who tested positive for HIV when she went to a public health clinic to confirm her pregnancy. She is due at any time, and while she should be joyous about the birth of her baby, she is grief-stricken that she won't live to see her child's tenth birthday, that her child also may have the disease and that her husband also may not be around to care for the child. At the beginning of my involvement with the AIDS epidemic, it seemed perfectly clear to me that no HIV-infected woman should become pregnant. I thought that no HIV-infected woman would want to have a baby either. I really didn't believe that an uninfected woman would want to have an infected man's child.

But I have learned that the desire for a baby is so enormous that many women choose to become pregnant in spite of the specter of disease. There are many reasons — to feel complete as a woman, to meet the expectations of their partner and others, because this is her last chance to leave something of herself behind when she realizes her life will be cut short, or because she's in denial about her own or her partner's illness and can't see the difficulties that could arise.

For some women, childbearing is the only joy left in a life filled with unhappiness, spouse abuse, poverty, drug use, racism and perhaps the loss of another child to AIDS. Or their religious beliefs or culture may bar them from using contraceptives or having an abortion, while childbearing is seen as the primary responsibility of women in the society.

It's estimated that an infected mother has about a 30 percent chance of transmitting AIDS to her unborn fetus. You may think that a 30 percent chance of having an infected baby is a high risk. Some women are more optimistic and see this as a 70 percent chance of having a healthy baby. As one HIV-infected woman said, "Those are the best odds I've heard since my diagnosis."

Because of the long-term ramifications of a woman with HIV disease giving birth, I strongly advise couples considering having children to be tested prior to pregnancy if they think there is any risk at all that they may have been exposed to HIV.

Consider the following scenarios:

- You've been using condoms with your partner, and now you want to get pregnant. Is it safe to stop using condoms? Maybe before you decide on whether you want a boy or a girl, you should both be tested for HIV.
- You're married and you want to have children. Should you be tested?
- What if you or your partner are HIV infected? Should you have a baby?
- What if during your pregnancy, you find out your partner is HIV infected?
- What if during your pregnancy, you find out you are HIV infected?
- If you are HIV infected, what are the chances your baby will be born infected as well?

If you and your partner decide to be tested before you get pregnant, here's what could happen:

- You and your partner may both test negative and if you want to have a baby, HIV disease is no problem for you or your baby.
- You are positive and your partner is negative. You need to take into account that you could infect your partner while having unprotected sex and that you could also pass on the virus to your baby. We can't accurately pinpoint which women are most apt to transmit the disease to the unborn fetus. But we are beginning to believe that if you are in the early stages with no symptoms of HIV disease, odds are better that the baby will be born uninfected. The longer you've had the virus and the more symptoms you manifest, the more likely that your baby will be born HIV infected. There's also the possibility that women who are being treated with drugs like AZT are less likely to pass on the virus to their babies. We don't have all the answers yet.

I know an HIV-infected woman who is now pregnant with her second baby. Her spouse is still negative and hadn't until recently understood that one day his wife will be dead and his children will be left with no mother. He will have the sole responsibility of caring for his children, one of whom may be doomed to a death sentence before the age of two.

- You could be negative and your partner could be positive. If you still want to have a baby with a father who is positive, you should understand that you could be infected at the same time you're getting pregnant because you won't be using a condom.

I find it difficult to recommend having unprotected sex at any time with an infected partner, but if you are determined, you could reduce your chances for getting infected by using a condom all of the time that you're not fertile. Stop using the condom *only* when you are ovulating, at the time of the month you are likely to conceive. Your doctor can help you determine the most fertile time of the month. Remember, an infected woman can infect her baby, so please use a condom for the rest of your pregnancy to help protect both you and your unborn child.

You could also consider artificial insemination, that is, using the semen from an HIV-negative donor. Make sure your doctor uses a legitimate donor bank, where proper testing ensures that the semen is from a healthy donor.

A bisexual man I know tested HIV positive before he got married. He told his wife he was bisexual and that he was HIV positive. They decided to have a child anyway. His wife is now pregnant and still tests negative for HIV. She believes she will remain so, even though she and her husband obviously have had, and maybe are still having, unprotected sex.

- You both test positive for HIV. You need to think not only about the risks of passing this virus on to your baby, but also about who will take care of the child when you and your partner are too ill to do so.

Remember Sherry and Stan from Chapter 1? Before they decided to have a baby, they came to me for testing. Both tested positive. Although Stan remained handsome and healthy after passing the virus on to his wife, Sherry is already dead. What would it have been like for Stan or Sherry's parents, who nursed their daughter in her final months, if she had had a baby? After the heart-wrenching experience of watching their only daughter die, they then would have had the responsibility of taking care of a grandchild who might have been infected, too.

Deciding whether to have a child or, if the law allows, whether to terminate the pregnancy is an excruciatingly difficult decision for a woman to make. Statistics show that about half the women who are HIV infected decide to have their babies.

Those opting for terminating the pregnancy may have a hard time finding a doctor to do this procedure. In these days when abortion laws are coming under fire, it is not easy to find gynecologists who will terminate a pregnancy. And those doctors who will perform abortions have the added complexity of dealing with HIV infection. Thus, many woman find it difficult to obtain an abortion if they are HIV infected, and it may cost them up to three times more to have the procedure done.

The HIV-Positive Baby: What Does It Mean?

If the mother is HIV positive, it means that she has (a) HIV virus and (b) antibodies to that virus. She can pass on the virus or the antibodies or both to her unborn baby. The baby may be born as follows:

- With no virus and no antibodies. This baby will be HIV negative and healthy.

- With no virus, but with antibodies. This baby is not HIV infected, but will test HIV positive because of the maternal antibodies. The baby will lose the maternal antibodies over a period of time and will then test HIV negative.
- With the virus, but no antibodies yet because of the window period. This baby will test negative initially, but will actually be infected and will later test positive.
- With the virus and antibodies. This baby is also infected with HIV disease and has only a small chance of surviving beyond the age of two.

During an infected infant's lifetime, he or she will be subjected to a variety of illnesses, including pneumonia, tuberculosis and painful thrush.

Because it's difficult to test for the virus, sometimes it takes up to 15 months before we know whether that baby is truly uninfected and healthy. Those 15 months of not knowing are terrible months for any parent to endure.

Some other tests are available, but they are not thoroughly reliable and don't always clarify the situation any earlier. (See Chapter 8 for more information on testing.)

During a recent lecture, I was approached by a woman who had questions about her daughter and grandson. Her daughter had been diagnosed with HIV infection when she delivered an HIV-positive infant. Now, the grandmother said, her daughter had just told her the baby was no longer HIV positive.

"I don't understand what this means," she said. "I think my daughter is trying to hide bad news from me."

"Your daughter is probably telling you the truth," I explained. The infant had probably lost the maternal antibodies and was not HIV infected. He is one of the fortunate 70 percent of children born to HIV-infected mothers who will not get AIDS. The grandmother was relieved to have her daughter's story validated, knowing that her grandson would be all right, yet her happiness was tainted by the bitter fact that her grandson would soon be motherless.

The Effects Of Pregnancy

At this time we don't know whether pregnancy will accelerate the progress of disease in an HIV-infected woman. Informal evidence suggests that it won't. We also don't know the full effect of HIV disease on the fetus. Many pregnant HIV-positive women are subject to other significant factors affecting their health, such as substance abuse, poor nutrition or poor prenatal care. These factors may contribute to complications during pregnancy and childbirth.

We also don't know what effects drugs such as AZT have on the pregnant woman and her baby. Until recently pregnant women were excluded from taking AZT because of the unknown effects of AZT on the fetus. At present we believe that the benefits of treating the mother outweigh the risk of complication for the fetus, and that AZT doesn't adversely affect the fetus. Additionally some of the drugs used to stop other infections in HIV-positive women are also being recommended for pregnant women. Again the reasoning is that the health of the mother is of prime importance. The fetus can't grow if the mother is dead.

We don't even know whether it is better to deliver babies of HIV-infected women by Caesarean section or by vaginal delivery. Which way is more effective in decreasing the risk of infecting the baby?

Even a mother's milk may not be safe from the scourge of this virus. There is some evidence to suggest that a baby born uninfected could later be infected by breast-feeding. The first time we understood this was when a mother, who was negative until getting a blood transfusion at the time of delivery, breast-fed her baby. That blood transfusion was infectious. The baby was negative at birth, but became HIV positive after nursing his newly infected mother. It is thought the baby got the virus through the breast milk. Other recent reports seem to verify this, and doctors now recommend that HIV-infected mothers should not breast-feed their babies.

In some countries, however, the risk of unsafe water and milk is higher than the risk of getting HIV disease from breast milk. So in Third World countries, mothers are still encouraged to breast-feed because the alternatives might be even more dangerous.

Artificial Insemination Or Egg Donor

Some women who want a child may not have a partner to father the baby or they may have a partner who is unable to father a child because of infertility, HIV infection or genetic diseases they don't want to pass on to the baby. These women may be candidates for artificial insemination using donated sperm.

Since the HIV test became available, regulated sperm banks now test donors. If you are considering artificial insemination, please make sure the sperm donor bank is doing at least the following to screen for HIV disease:

- Screening donors by history so that anyone at high risk will be eliminated.
- Conducting an HIV screening test at the time of donation.
- Storing the sperm by freezing for six months before use, so that the donor can be retested. If the donor still tests negative, the sperm can be used. As with blood donors, because of the window period, these safeguards are not 100 percent risk free.

If a woman wants to be artificially inseminated with her mate's sperm, then the couple should be tested in the same manner as prior to a normal pregnancy.

Women who are infertile and receive an egg donated by another woman should make sure their infertility doctor has tested the donor prior to implanting the donor egg or oocyte. However, unlike the sperm, the egg cannot be kept for six months to allow the donor to be retested. But another new test, the PCR, is now being explored and may be useful in this situation. For increased safeguards, the donor can have both the HIV test and a PCR probe done. The PCR test costs about $150.

Pregnancy And HIV — A Troubling Issue

One of the worst stories I have ever heard was about a pregnant, desperately ill IV drug-using woman who was admitted to a county hospital. When she was diagnosed as having AIDS, she refused treatment. However, the decision wasn't legally hers to make. Because she was pregnant and there was a fetus to consider, she was placed on life-saving devices without her permission just to keep her and the fetus alive until the birth of her child. She stayed hooked up to a respirator even though she became comatose.

The baby was born alive. The mother died. I don't know if the baby had AIDS or not. But this story raises all sorts of medical and ethical questions for me.

Who did we need to take care of here? The mother or the fetus? Who should bear the enormous cost of the pregnancy and illness? Who will take care of this infant who has about a 30 percent chance of having AIDS?

HIV-Infected Mothers

HIV-infected mothers have special problems. They often neglect their own medical care in favor of their children's needs.

I put the question to Audrey, one of my patients, about what concerned her most about her disease.

"My children," she exclaimed, without hesitation. "What will happen to them? Their daddy is already dead. I'm in the dying process and they are teenagers struggling with their own issues." Tears welled up in her eyes. "I worry about my children."

Audrey had acquired the virus from her husband of 18 years. He had developed a drug habit and had actually moved out of the house. A year after his death, Audrey found the courage to be tested. She is now being treated with AZT and is working to support her two teenage children. We often exchange our experiences of the joys and difficulties of rearing teenagers. Her children's problems, however, are profound — they've had to deal with a parent addicted to and killed by drugs and the dying process of the other parent.

How do they cope with the challenges of growing up? I sit here and cry for Audrey's children as I write this, and cry for the millions of children in this world who will be born to parents affected with this curse. It seems they inherit the curse too.

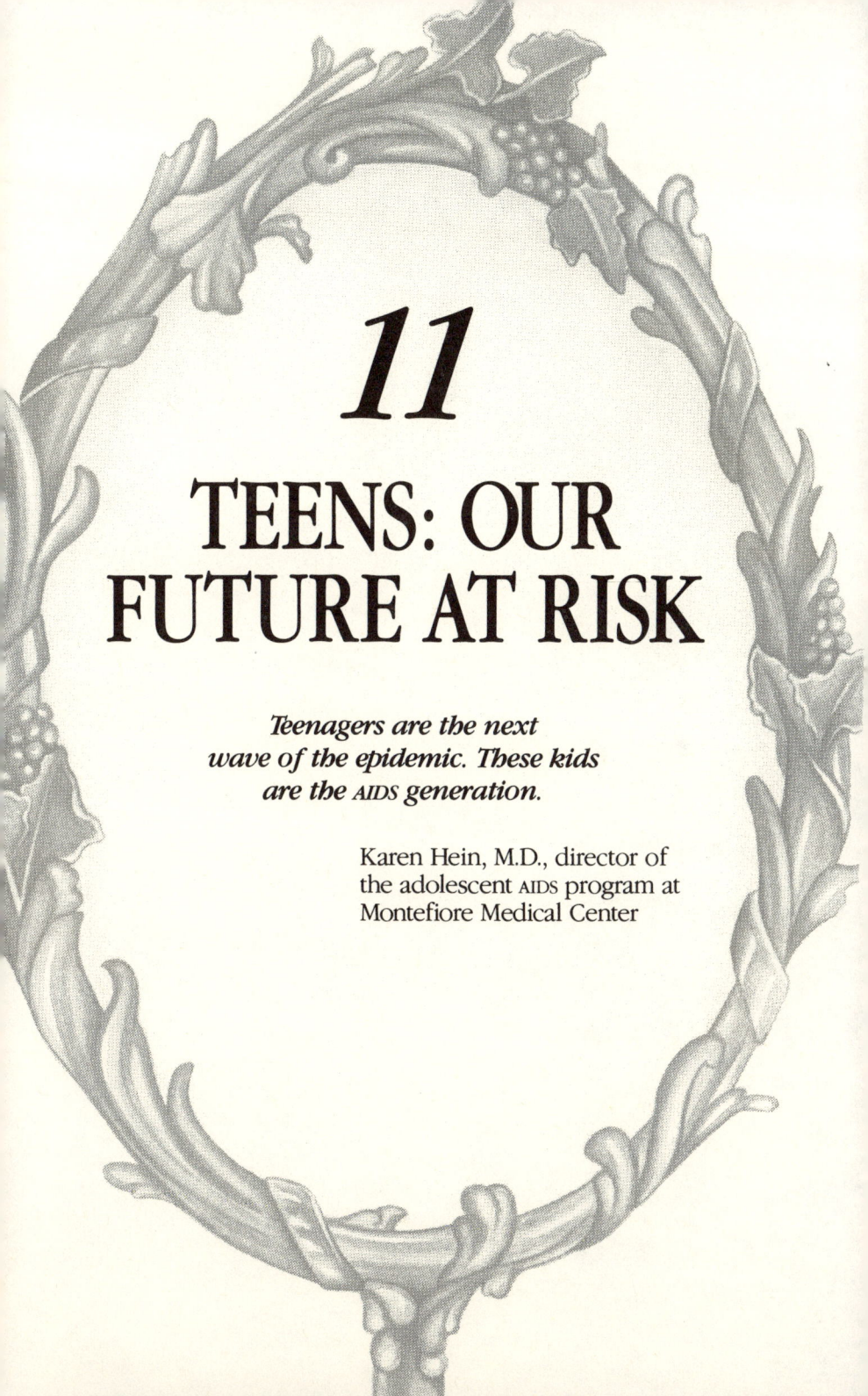

11

TEENS: OUR FUTURE AT RISK

*Teenagers are the next
wave of the epidemic. These kids
are the AIDS generation.*

Karen Hein, M.D., director of
the adolescent AIDS program at
Montefiore Medical Center

A 14-year-old patient of mine who was recently discharged from a drug and alcohol program told me she had had sex "just a few times" in the past, as far as she could remember. Nadine couldn't recall if her partners had used condoms; she couldn't recall if she enjoyed having sex. She couldn't even recall if she had been high at the time. Nadine and other girls her age are not only at risk for teenage pregnancy, alcohol and drug-related problems, but are also in the category of highest risk for getting AIDS.

I feel terribly helpless when I think about Nadine. By the time we have the opportunity to rehabilitate her — she's an intelligent youngster with a potentially bright future — she could either be dead with the AIDS virus or dying. She could possibly have one or more HIV-infected children. She could have infected several men also, who in turn, could have infected several other women, who could, in turn, have had several HIV-infected children. The dreadful possibilities are endless.

I've often wondered if Nadine hears my advice about safe sex and if it makes any difference to her. How do we get through to these kids? Can we? If we don't, their future — and ours — is dismal.

The fact is the HIV epidemic threatens the very existence of the next generation. The number of teenage AIDS cases doubles each year. If you think I'm catastrophizing, consider how quickly the estimated numbers of people contracting the disease are being revised upward. This virus is spreading rapidly around the world, and teenagers like Nadine are both promoting it and victims of it.

Many mothers who are unable to talk to their teenagers themselves ask me to counsel their children. A new patient of mine, Lillian, a recently divorced woman in her late 30s, brought her teenager in for counseling.

I respected and admired Lillian for her concern about Emily and was pleased for the opportunity to discuss sexuality, abstinence and safe sex with the girl before she became sexually active. However, when I asked Lillian, the mother, if she was practicing safe sex, her mouth dropped open.

"I never thought about it happening to me," she responded. I was amazed — this from a single, sexually active intelligent woman.

Young People And AIDS

Many teenagers think that AIDS simply will not affect them. After all, they're young, healthy and certainly not vulnerable to fatal diseases. But because they are still experimenting with sex and are likely to have unprotected sex with multiple partners, they are our highest risk group for AIDS.

Public health offficials do not yet have a good grasp of how many teens have been infected because they are unable to do widespread testing.

It is important to understand that AIDS may go undiag-
nosed in young people because they look and feel healthy
for many years. Health officials believe that as many as a
third or more of the people who have died of AIDS in this
country acquired the virus when they were teenagers.

We *do* know that AIDS has become the seventh leading
cause of death in people ages 15 to 24. And we know that
three to four out of every 1,000 teenagers who were
tested when applying for the Job Corps in 1991 were HIV
positive. The studies of adolescents applying to the military have shown a slightly lower incidence, but these statistics are slightly skewed since IV drug users and homosexuals are barred from the military and probably would
not apply.

Between 1987 and 1991, researchers at the Children's
National Medical Center in Washington, D.C., tested
blood samples from all patients ages 13 to 19 years who
received care for any reason at the Center. In 1987, 1 out
of 400 male adolescents tested were found to be positive.
By 1991, the number had risen to 1 in 80. It is predicted
that very soon it may be 1 in 50.

Three million teenagers are infected by genital warts
or other sexually transmitted diseases, including chlamydia, herpes, syphilis and gonorrhea. We know that people
with a sexually transmitted disease are at higher risk for
becoming infected with HIV. And because the AIDS virus is
more easily transmitted to women than to men, adolescent
females are at extremely high risk.

Consider teenage runaways, living on the streets, sell-
ing their bodies for money and drugs, having what we call
survival sex. These youngsters may never see adulthood
because of AIDS. The cure is probably years away and the
young people who contract AIDS now will probably not see
it in their lifetime.

The average number of sex partners young people will have by the time they graduate from college is five. Even though they may believe in monogamy, their definition is different. It's actually serial monogamy — they have sex exclusively with one person for a while and then go on to the next partner.

A survey of students and frequency of condom use showed that only 25 percent used condoms every single time they had intercourse. Thirty-seven percent rarely or never used them.

Teenagers have what we call "scared sex." First they have sex, then they get scared afterward that they may be infected with AIDS or may be pregnant. The fear of pregnancy motivates many young women to use birth control devices — such as birth control pills, diaphragms or sponges — but not necessarily condoms.

Teens make comments like, "AIDS has me scared about sex," but they still don't use condoms. They may have intellectual awareness about AIDS, but they don't apply it to their own behavior.

There are a number of reasons why young people aren't listening. If we talk about AIDS and death, teens become so terrified they can't hear the message. It's too frightening for them to be in touch with their own mortality. Equating unprotected sex with death is the ultimate truth and they know it, but rather than change their behavior, many deny it can happen to them.

No One's Disease

Once again, AIDS becomes somebody else's disease. Women think it's a disease of men; African-Americans prefer to think this is a white person's disease; straight people think it's a gay or IV drug user disease; young people think it's a disease of adulthood. Psychological defensiveness contributes greatly to the tragedy of AIDS.

Teenagers tend to think AIDS is a disease of adults because of its long incubation period. Most of them who
have friends with the virus have yet to see them with
full-blown AIDS, since the horror of it won't be evident
until years later.

While Magic Johnson is certainly reaching more young
ears than anyone previously has on the subject of AIDS, I
can't help but question his impact. He himself still looks
and feels healthy; his wife and child are not affected and
Magic keeps on smiling, playing basketball and appearing
to enjoy his life to the max.

Denial runs rampant among college-age students as
well. I'm reminded of Mark, a handsome, intelligent 19-
year-old, who was a premedical student living with his
lover, a man he knew to be HIV positive. They didn't practice safe sex because Mark thought AIDS could never
happen to him. He knew all about it. His lover was HIV
positive, but Mark's denial was so great it cost him his
life. He was tested and found positive. It was agonizing
for me to tell him his results.

How do we counsel young HIV-positive people about
what to do with the rest of their lives? Mark was asymptomatic, healthy looking and only recently infected. Should
he go to medical school with the hope that by some mir-
acle he'd escape AIDS? Or was there hope that a cure
would be found by the time he completed medical school?
Or should he refrain from the rigors of an intensive educational program and enjoy the rest of his life?

Mark decided to go to medical school, and he taught me
a valuable lesson: Knowledge about this virus doesn't protect anyone from getting it.

So what do we teach young people? What are the messages we need to tell them? The messages can vary, depending who they are, how old they are and how they
view their own sexuality.

For most, we should be giving the message of abstinence.

Most of us who grew up in the '40s, '50s and early '60s accepted the idea that sex belonged solely in marriage. The sexual revolution exploded that belief. But the AIDS epidemic is slowly bringing back the age of chastity. It takes a while for standards to change, but I'm beginning to discover more and more teenagers who say they won't have sex until they get married. Peer pressure affirming that it is okay not to have sex is starting to build.

Recently, while I was addressing an auditorium filled with high school students, I was reminded to teach the lesson of abstinence. I had been talking about safe sex, giving explicit instructions, thinking I was being "cool," answering questions such as "Are flavored condoms safe?", explaining exactly how to put on a condom, how to take it off and how to dispose of it.

Then one young woman raised her hand and asked, "Dr. Sack, what's wrong with waiting until you're married to have sex? You keep talking about safer sex, why don't you talk about abstinence?"

At first, the audience snickered. Some of them even booed at the word abstinence. I knew at once that I had done the teenagers a terrible disservice. I'd forgotten to tell them that abstinence is the only safe solution. Even I, a physician and AIDS educator, was giving them the wrong message.

I congratulated the young woman on bringing the best suggestion of all, and told the audience that she deserved a round of applause for her clear thinking. At first only one student joined me as I began applauding, but then others joined in until eventually half the audience showed their support.

Teenagers need permission, not only from an authority like myself, but from their peers to choose abstinence as an option. Even kids who have had sex can become abstinent. (They call themselves the "born-again virgins.") We should let them know we support their decision.

Miami psychologist Suzanne Keeley believes strongly that abstinence is not just about morality. It is also about optimal health. "It's good medically because it's in young people's best interests," she says. "In the past, they had to worry about venereal diseases and unwanted pregnancy, but now there's AIDS. What was dangerous then is deadly now, and the message that sex is okay is killing our kids."

Teenagers at one school were asked to write down 101 ways they could make love without "doing it." Here are some of their suggestions:

- Tell the other person you love them.
- Make the other person feel important and respected.
- Trust one another.
- Talk to each other.
- Whisper something nice into the other's ear.
- Flirt with each other.
- Find out what makes the other happy.
- Dedicate a song on the radio.
- Find out what makes the other sad.
- Share an ice cream cone.

(I think these teenagers can offer adults many pointers about the importance of being intimate rather than sexual.)

How do teens just say no to sex? There are many ways to say no, and here are a few suggestions:

- "I'm just not ready for it yet."
- "I don't want to."
- "It may seem right for you, but I'm not going to do it until I'm sure this is the right thing for me."
- "I care about you, but the responsibility that comes with sex is too much for me right now."
- "I've made a decision not to have sex until I get married, and that's a good decision for me."
- "I think that sex is wrong outside of marriage."

- "I'm afraid of pregnancy, AIDS and sexually transmitted diseases. Let's find other ways of being romantic."

A Virgin's Story

Heather, a young patient of mine, told me that she has chosen to remain a virgin until marriage because of the AIDS epidemic.

"Before we get married, I'll ask my boyfriend to have an AIDS test," she said. "I hope to think with my head, not with my body, so that I can remain healthy for myself, my husband and my future children. Sex would be nice, but I'm not willing to give up my health for it."

The Fact Is, Some Teens Do It

No matter how much we encourage abstinence, there are teens who will have sex. I know, because many of them come to talk to me about it. Very few of them, incidentally, are enjoying sex. They ask me questions like:

"Dr. Sack, is it always going to hurt?"

"Dr. Sack, is this what it's all about?"

"It doesn't seem like in the movies or in the books."

"Sex was okay, but I never had an orgasm and don't even know how to have an orgasm."

"I've had sex with a guy who I thought loved me and now he's dumped me and I feel terrible."

One 15-year-old, who had had many sex partners, said, "Dr. Sack, I'm so confused. I don't know why I'm having sex." Very rarely have teenagers talked to me about the pleasures of sex.

I'm well aware that I can't convert all of my sexually active teenagers into "abstainers." The most I can do is discuss my view of healthy sexuality, the dangers of sex and how to protect themselves.

I'm also concerned that our message about sex being safe with a condom gives a false sense of security, leading teenagers and others to believe that condoms are 100 percent safe. In fact, some people compare using a condom to driving a car at 95 mph around a deadly curve — you feel as if you're safe because you have on your seatbelt.

These condom nonbelievers point out that there's a high pregnancy rate among people using condoms. And if people can get pregnant only during a narrow window of time each month, consider the odds when one can contract AIDS 365 days of the year.

I believe that condoms can be fairly safe if they are used correctly and used all of the time.

We know that adults are often embarrassed to talk about sex. It's even more awkward for young people to talk about it. When I begin to talk about safer sex, teens giggle, blush and squirm. They may not talk about it, but embarrassment doesn't stop teens from having sex.

Sometimes they're too embarrassed to buy condoms for themselves, so their mothers buy them. I've heard of mothers who buy boxes of condoms, leave them in the closet and then tell the teenagers, "I won't count if you don't count."

If teens are not mature enough to buy their own condoms, I wonder if they're mature enough to have sex. But it's really not my place to judge, and I'm pleased at least that they're reducing their risks by wearing condoms.

Developing The Dialogue

Teenagers are constantly being reminded about AIDS and know they are at risk. But because they are sexually inexperienced, they are embarrassed to talk to their partner about sex. As parents and educators, we can help them by developing the dialogue.

For example, they can begin a conversation with their sex partner by saying, "I need to talk to you about something that's important to both of us. This is hard for me to do, and I'm embarrassed, but I think we need to talk about AIDS and safer sex." Or, "I've been hearing a lot about AIDS recently, and I worry about it. Here's what I think we should do to protect ourselves."

Yet all around them, teens receive other messages about sex. Adults sell products with sex, use sex in movies, television and music — then we tell teens to "just say no." No wonder they are conflicted and have a difficult time making decisions about sex.

Let's find a way to spread the message to teens that they are the future, our hope for survival. What kind of future will our planet have if our young people are killed by this virus? Let's empower them to start thinking about how they can protect themselves.

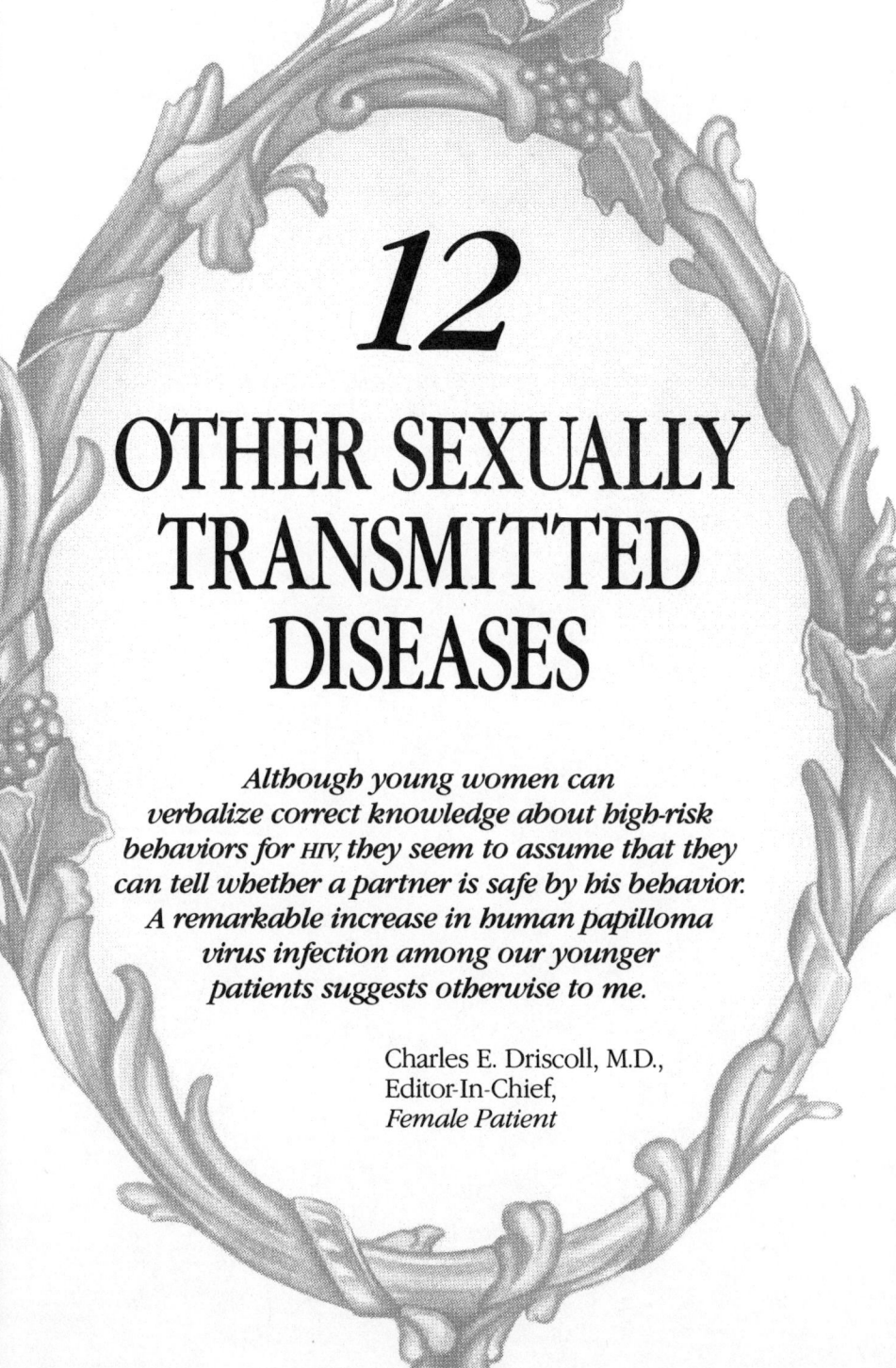

12

OTHER SEXUALLY TRANSMITTED DISEASES

*Although young women can
verbalize correct knowledge about high-risk
behaviors for* HIV, *they seem to assume that they
can tell whether a partner is safe by his behavior.
A remarkable increase in human papilloma
virus infection among our younger
patients suggests otherwise to me.*

Charles E. Driscoll, M.D.,
Editor-In-Chief,
Female Patient

A month ago, a patient who has been married for six months came to my office with a problem she couldn't discuss with her family or friends. Leslie felt as if she were being stifled by her husband. He wanted to treat her like a princess and didn't want her to work because he made enough money. He didn't want her to make her own friends because he liked to spend all the time he could with her. And he always wanted to make love.

Leslie thought something was wrong with her because she couldn't always have an orgasm. We talked a long time about her needs, her feelings of self-worth and about the fact that she didn't always have to have an orgasm in order to be a good wife.

Then Paul, her husband, came to see me. He had a rash on his penis, he said, and wanted some cream. His rash was herpes. He told me that just before getting married, he "made love to another woman." He didn't use a condom because "she looked clean." This woman had gone to see her doctor, and had called Paul the next week to inform him that he should see his doctor. He didn't go to the doctor because at first he saw nothing unusual. Now, he didn't remember the woman's name, didn't have her phone number and had tried to forget the telephone call because he was married and didn't intend to "make love to anyone else."

We discussed herpes and how it was transmitted, and the fact that he may have contracted other sexually transmitted diseases from the same "clean-looking lady." I convinced Paul to have an HIV test.

Then I had a second conversation with his wife. Paul had told Leslie about the other woman and the herpes, and, understandably, she was afraid of getting herpes from him and transmitting it to her future children.

She was also afraid of the results of his AIDS test.

"This is terrible for me," she said. "How can I live knowing that either Paul or I may have AIDS?" We talked about her fears, and I assured Leslie that the chances were small, but I had done the test on her husband to be 100 percent certain.

"Dr. Sack, he won't come and get the results," she said. "He doesn't want to hear the news if he tested positive."

I was perplexed. "What about you?" I asked.

"I don't know what to do," she replied.

"I know what you should do," I said. "Until you both know the results of his test, you should ask Paul to wear a condom."

"Dr. Sack," Leslie said, "he won't."

As I write this, Paul has not yet visited me for his results. What kind of person is this, I wonder, who loves a woman enough to marry her, who is so possessive of her that he takes away her freedom to be herself, who makes love to another woman on the eve of their marriage and then won't wear a condom to protect his spouse?

Leslie feels — and acts — powerless. Until we as a society teach women to say no to unprotected sex, even with their husbands, this epidemic will go on relentlessly. And other sexually transmitted diseases will continue to spread unchecked.

Kevin, a teenage patient of mine, has a father dying of AIDS. His father's illness has profoundly affected Kevin, so I was quite surprised when he came in asking to be checked for chlamydia. He explained that his girlfriend had chlamydia.

He shook his head when I asked if they had been using condoms.

"Why not?" I asked.

"I figured Barbara was clean and didn't have AIDS," he said. "I thought we were monogamous."

"But?"

"Well, she did catch chlamydia from someone else, but I still don't think she has AIDS," he explained.

When I tried to convince Kevin to use condoms for protection against AIDS and other sexually transmitted diseases (STDs), he told me didn't like using condoms.

When I asked what he was using for contraceptives, he replied, "Nothing."

"What if Barbara gets pregnant?" I countered.

"Oh, Dr. Sack, please don't say that. That would be terrible for me. My last girlfriend needed an abortion and I never got over the trauma of that!"

People's reluctance to change — to do what they know is good for them — shows that we really have a long way to go before we will end the spread of AIDS and other STDs, and decrease the rate of unwanted pregnancies.

HIV And STDS: A Lot In Common

Sexually transmitted diseases is a broad term that refers to infections acquired from having sex with an unprotected person. STDs are sometimes referred to as venereal diseases (VD). There are about 20 different STDs and they are spread from person to person by close physical contact during vaginal, anal or oral sex. STDs can be spread from woman to man, man to woman, woman to woman or man to man.

According to the Centers for Disease Control, here's how the more common STDs stack up: More than four million American men and women get chlamydia each year; three million get genital warts; one million get gonorrhea and 500,000 get genital herpes. You may wonder why you need to know about sexually transmitted diseases when HIV disease appears to be more serious. The truth is, if you have an STD, you are at higher risk for acquiring and spreading HIV disease. In fact, some studies suggest that your risk for acquiring HIV increases 100 times simply by having an STD. That's because the ulcerlike sores associated with many of the STDs offer a perfect entry point for HIV.

Additionally both AIDS and STDs have in common the fact that unprotected sexual intercourse is the easiest way to be infected. The frightening part is that STDs are increasing in spite of massive education and information campaign efforts urging safer sex.

How STDs Make Their Rounds

All sexually transmitted bacteria and viruses need to live in warm, moist places. The vagina, urethra, rectum and mouth are perfect "homes."

Sexually transmitted diseases, such as herpes or genital warts, can be contracted by kissing, caressing or being in close contact with infected areas. Some diseases are passed only through sexual intercourse. Some STDs are just an annoyance. Some are more dangerous: If left untreated, they can cause permanent damage such as blindness, brain damage or infertility. HIV disease is the most serious since it causes death.

Many STDs — including AIDS, chlamydia, genital warts, gonorrhea, herpes and syphilis — can be passed on from a mother to her unborn baby, sometimes causing severe complications, even death.

Genital warts can lead to precancerous conditions and an increased chance for cancer of the cervix. And some sexually transmitted diseases, such as chlamydia and gonorrhea, can cause infertility in both men and women.

Some sexually transmitted diseases such as AIDS and herpes cannot be cured.

Questions And Answers About STDs

Q. Do STDs cause special problems for women?

A. Yes. They can be harder to diagnose. There may be no signs or the signs are inside the body where symptoms are not easily observed. A woman can have an STD for a long time without knowing it. In the meantime, there can be damage leading to ectopic pregnancies and infertility. Also many STDs can be transmitted from an infected mother to her baby during pregnancy or at birth, causing, in some cases, permanent damage or even death to the infant.

Q. Do STDs cause AIDS?

A. No, they are not a direct cause of AIDS, but HIV is more easily transmitted among people who have other STDs which cause genital sores, such as herpes and syphilis.

Anyone with an STD should have tests for other common STDs, as well as an HIV test. When people have one STD, they're likely to have other STDs as well. Similarly, HIV-infected people should be tested for other STDs.

Q. What are some signs of STDs?

A. The symptoms of STDs are different for men and women. Here are some of the more *common signs in women:*

- Unusual vaginal discharge and odor.
- Pain in lower abdomen.

- Burning, itching or pain in vagina.
- Unusual vaginal bleeding.

For men, the signs are:

- "Drip" or discharge from penis.
- Pain in the testes.

Both men and women may have these symptoms as well:

- Sores, bumps, ulcer or blisters on the genitals.
- Burning while urinating.
- Sore throat.
- No symptoms.

Q. What if I'm diagnosed with an STD?
A. If you are diagnosed with an STD, you must:

1. Tell your partner(s) because they might be infected and should be tested and treated. If you have a problem doing this, the public health department will help you through the partner notification program.
2. Avoid having sex while you're being treated.
3. Follow your doctor's instructions, complete all of your medication and go for follow-up visits.

Q. What are the symptoms and treatment of the most common STDs?

A. Here's a brief description of each of the more common STDs:

Chlamydia is the most common sexually transmitted disease in the United States today. Chlamydia is a bacterial infection and is a dangerous disease because it is often silent until it has caused great damage. That is, most people don't know they have *chlamydia* until it has caused painful and permanent damage to the sex and pelvic organs. This damage can leave both men and women unable to have children.

There may be noticeable signs within one to four weeks after having sex with someone who is infected. But 80 percent of women and 10 percent of men have no symptoms. In men, chlamydia can infect the urethra and the testicles, causing a discharge or crusting at the tip of the penis.

Women may only discover the disease after their male partners begin to show symptoms, or if their doctor finds it during an examination. In women, the disease first invades the cervix, then travels into the uterus and into the fallopian tubes and ovaries. There may be some discharge from the vagina, or pain in the lower part of the abdomen, as well as pain or burning when urinating. Women may also experience pain on having sex, abnormal vaginal bleeding and bleeding after sexual intercourse. Often it is only detected after developing into pelvic inflammatory disease (PID). This is an infection which, if untreated, can cause great damage to the reproductive organs of a woman, thus making her infertile.

A mother with chlamydia can pass it on to her child during childbirth. Many of these babies will suffer from eye infections and pneumonia.

The good news is that chlamydia can be cured by antibiotics. Sex partners must also be treated or the disease can be passed on again and again.

Herpes simplex is a common, contagious and incurable virus that causes recurrent small, usually painful sores on the mouth or genital area. Signs of herpes are usually apparent within 2 to 10 days after sex with an infected person.

The symptoms may include a burning sensation or pain when urinating; pain in the buttocks, genitals or legs; or a discharge from the vagina. Women may have sores on the inner and outer lips of the vagina or urethra, and men may have sores on the penis or scrotum. Often a woman may have sores in the cervix that go undetected.

The small sores generally fill up with fluid, then these blisters scab over and heal. Sores can spring up in crops, lasting for one to two weeks, then healing in three weeks. Other symptoms include fever, fatigue, headaches and large lymph nodes in the groin. Once the sores heal, however, the virus goes into hiding in the cells close to the area where the sores originated. At this point, the infected person doesn't usually pass the infection on to others, but can.

Some people experience only one herpes outbreak, while others may have repeated active outbreaks with recurring symptoms. Usually, one is only infectious when there are symptoms. When the sores recur, they are usually much less severe than the first time and they heal more quickly. Pain, however, is still common, and appears to be more severe in females than in males.

We don't know why herpes affects individuals so differently. Some may have outbreaks 12 times a year; others only once. For some, the outbreaks occur less frequently as the years pass. We do know that people whose immune systems are not working properly, as with HIV disease, get severe herpes outbreaks more frequently.

One of the problems with herpes is that if a pregnant woman has herpes at the time she delivers the baby, the baby can get herpes. This causes serious, sometimes life-threatening illnesses in newborns. The effects on the baby or fetus are worse if it's an infection contracted during the pregnancy. To protect herself and the fetus, a pregnant woman who has never had herpes should use a condom if she has a sex partner who has or had herpes.

Pregnant women with herpes should consult with their doctors, who will want to follow their pregnancies closely. Before the baby is born, the doctor will need to determine the risk of transmitting the virus to the child during the birth. He or she may opt for a Caesarean section delivery.

Herpes is diagnosed by the physician, who takes a sample of the fluid from the blister and has a culture of the virus grown. There are no cures or vaccines for herpes. Medicine can merely minimize the severity and frequency of the herpes outbreaks with a relatively new drug, Acyclovir (Zovirax). This is an anti-viral agent and is sometimes given to people with herpes daily to prevent outbreaks.

As with other STDs, latex condoms and nonoxynol-9 help reduce the spread of herpes. If the herpes virus is located in parts of the body a condom won't cover — for example, the buttocks — the area should be covered either with plastic wrap or a bandaid. Skin-to-skin contact should be avoided.

- *Cold sores* on the lips are caused by the herpes virus, usually Herpes Type I. Genital sores are usually Herpes Type II. Cold sores are actually herpes and can be transmitted by kissing. A cold sore on the lip can be transmitted to the sex partner's genital area through oral sex. The virus can also be transmitted to other parts of the body by touching the lip or genital sore with the hand, then touching other parts of the body with the hand.
- *Genital or venereal warts* are caused by the human papilloma virus (HPV). This virus is very contagious. These growths appear in, around or on the sex organs of both men and women. Some of the growths are flat, some are round bumps and some look like heads of cauliflowers. Warts may appear within three weeks to three months after having sex with someone who is infected. Some women develop warts inside the vagina where they can't be seen. They can also occur in or around the anus.

In men they occur on the penis or sometimes on the scrotum or around the anus.

Besides being visible, the warts sometimes cause symptoms of itching and burning. If the warts are not removed, they can grow into large masses that are hard to clear up.

Women with genital warts should have them treated before they become pregnant because some of the treatments are not safe during pregnancy. Genital warts can get so big during pregnancy that they can interfere with the birth of the baby. They can also be transmitted to the newborn. Infants of mothers with genital warts can develop warts on their vocal cords.

Genital warts can be cured, but they usually don't disappear by themselves. Both sex partners should be treated. Sometimes the doctor will paint them with medicine, causing them to fall off. Some are frozen or burned off. Some are removed surgically or with laser treatment. Sometimes they return, requiring periodic medical exams and follow-ups. These follow-ups are essential, as all types of genital warts may lead to cancer.

Gonorrhea is also known by other names, including clap, drip or GC. The disease is caused by a bacteria called *gonococcus.*

Gonorrhea usually shows up two to 21 days after having sex with an infected person. Most women, and many men, don't have symptoms for a while. Meanwhile, the bacteria is working its way from the cervix into the uterus and fallopian tubes, and ultimately throughout the pelvis.

Women may feel pain or a burning sensation when urinating, or notice a yellow discharge from the vagina. There may be bleeding between periods, pain in the pelvic area and fever.

Men will usually have symptoms from two to seven days after being infected. A man will experience pain when urinating and notice a discharge from the tip of his penis. The skin around the urethra can also become red and irritated. Sores found in the anus and rectum cause painful bowel movements and pus. Both men and women can get gonorrhea in their throat, making swallowing painful.

Untreated, gonorrhea can cause pelvic inflammatory disease and infertility, or it could spread throughout the bloodstream and the whole body, causing serious conditions such as infections of the heart, joints and lining of the brain. People can die from gonorrhea if left untreated.

To detect gonorrhea, the doctor collects a small amount of fluid from the penis or vagina. This is sent to a lab to be cultured. Gonorrhea is curable with antibiotics most of the time. But there are now strains of the disease which are resistant to antibiotics.

Gonorrhea can be passed on from the mother to the baby, usually causing infection of the eye, throat, lungs or skin of the newborn. This is not usually life-threatening if treated immediately.

Pelvic inflammatory disease (PID) is an infection of a woman's pelvic and sex organs — uterus, fallopian tubes and ovaries. Chlamydia and gonorrhea are the two main STDs that cause PID. Many women are unaware that they have PID infection, and it can spread and cause painful and permanent damage to their sex organs. One in five women who have had PID cannot have children. The more times that a woman has had PID, the more likely that she will be unable to have children.

Still more dangerous for the woman with PID is that if she becomes pregnant, the fetus may lodge in her fallopian tubes instead of the uterus. Called an ectopic or tubal pregnancy, this can be very serious, even life-threatening and may require surgery.

Syphilis has been known since Biblical times and is caused by a bacteria called *treponema pallidum*. A newly infected person may notice symptoms from 1 to 12 weeks after having sex with an infected partner. Most men with syphilis do notice symptoms, but many women don't. There may be one or more sores that look like small pimples, and they may be small or large. These sores usually do not hurt. They can be found in the penis, scrotum, labia, vagina, mouth, throat, fingers, breasts and anus. These sores, found at the site of the initial infection, are called chancres and are highly infectious.

Even without treatment, a chancre heals and completely disappears within four to six weeks, but this does not mean the disease has gone away.

The infected person enters the second stage of the disease. From two to 12 weeks after the sore disappears, a skin rash usually appears. It may cover the whole body or appear in only a few areas. Sometimes people feel as if they have the flu. The rash and the flu symptoms eventually disappear, but again, the disease hasn't gone away. Instead it enters the latent or resting stage.

After a period of time, the disease enters a third stage, called tertiary syphilis. In this stage, the nervous system, heart and blood vessels are infected. Syphilis can also infect the brain and spinal cord, damaging nerves and causing difficulty with walking, loss of bladder control, blindness, heart disease and brain damage.

A woman with syphilis can transmit it to her baby during pregnancy. Syphilis may cause a miscarriage or severe birth defects in the child.

Syphilis is diagnosed either from taking fluid from the original lesion or through a blood test. Syphilis is usually treatable with antibiotics, including penicillin.

Hepatitis B is caused by a virus that attacks the liver. It can be passed from one person to another by intimate contact, especially during sex, or when needles are shared during drug use. It is also found in contaminated blood and can be transmitted by a pregnant woman to her unborn baby. Symptoms include loss of weight, weakness, nausea, vomiting, pain in the stomach and the yellowing of the skin or of the white part of the eye, called jaundice.

To test for hepatitis B, a blood sample is sent by the physician to a lab to be examined. There is no treatment for hepatitis B, but most people will recover after a month or so. Occasionally, the disease will cause severe liver damage and even death. There is a vaccine available that will prevent illness from hepatitis B. Children, adolescents, healthcare workers and anyone at risk are urged to be vaccinated.

Q. How can I learn more about my own body, my own anatomy?

A. You can check yourself for any signs or symptoms that might indicate the presence of a sexually transmitted disease. Only a physician can make a proper diagnosis, but a careful check of your genital area and that of your partner may help you identify an STD so that you can take the steps to get treated.

You might want to use a mirror and position it so that you can see the entire genital area. Above your vagina is soft, fatty tissue called the mons pubis. Your pubic hair grows on the mons and between your legs on the fleshy area on either side of your vagina called the outer lips or labia majora.

Start your examination by spreading your pubic hair apart with your fingers, and carefully look for any bumps, blisters or warts on the skin.

A genital wart may look like warts you've seen on other parts of your body. They may first appear very small, and then develop into fleshy, cauliflowerlike appearances. Some warts are hard to see, but if you feel any bumpy growth, have it checked.

Examine the area covered by your pubic hair, and the outer lips of your vagina, and then spread the lips apart and take a look inside your inner lips, the hairless flaps of skin called the labia minora.

At the top of your inner lips, below the mons, is the clitoris. Your inner lips are attached to the underside of the clitoris, and right below the clitoris is an opening for your urinary tract and urethra. And below your urethra is your vagina. Take a close look at your clitoris, urinary

and vaginal openings, again looking for any bumps, blisters, sores or warts.

Some signs of sexually transmitted diseases may appear
in your vagina and your cervix, out of view, but you may
have a discharge.

While most women normally have some vaginal discharge, the discharge caused by an STD is thicker, has a
color — usually either greenish or yellow — and sometimes has an odor.

You should encourage your male partner to do a genital
examination as well. Or you can examine him yourself.
Start by examining the head of the penis from the urinary
opening down to where it extends just above the shaft.
The top or head of the penis contains the urinary opening
or urethra. If the man is not circumcised, he has a foreskin
which needs to be pulled back to examine the entire head
of the penis. Carefully look for bumps, sores, blisters or
warts on the skin. Some sexually transmitted diseases
cause a drip or discharge from the penis. This drip may be
thick, yellow, watery or slight.

After you've examined the head of the penis, move
down to the part of the penis called the shaft and look for
the same signs, then go on to the base, the very bottom of
the shaft where the pubic hair begins. At the base, try to
separate the pubic hair with your fingers so you can get
a good look at the skin underneath.

Underneath the penis are two sacs called the scrotum,
which enclose the testicles. The scrotum should also be
checked for any signs or symptoms.

If you find any signs or symptoms of STDs, please check
with your doctor.

Q. How can I prevent STD infections?

A. The only way to guarantee that you won't get an STD
is not to have sexual intercourse. Otherwise, reducing
your risk of getting an STD is the same as reducing your
risk of getting AIDS. You can start by having an uninfected,

faithful partner. The more people you have sex with, the more risky sex becomes.

And you can make safe choices, opting for outercourse (sex that doesn't include intercourse), which is generally safe except for the possibility of spreading genital warts or herpes through close contact. And always wear a latex condom with spermicidal jelly.

If you avoid one sexually transmitted disease, you can avoid them all.

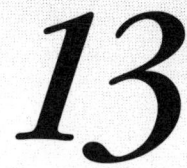

SAFETY OF THE HEALTHCARE SETTING: TWO SIDES OF THE COIN

Our challenge lies in addressing the justifiable concerns about HIV transmission in the healthcare setting while keeping in mind that the global HIV epidemic remains largely spread by sexual contact and injecting drug use.

Mary E. Chamberland, M.D., and
David M. Bell, M.D., Centers for
Disease Control, Atlanta

*T*he safety of the healthcare setting is of utmost importance to all — but in sheer numbers, particularly to women. Of the seven million people employed in hospitals and healthcare services in this country, 75 percent are women. And on any given day, the majority of patients in a hospital are women. Two-thirds of all surgeries are performed on women. Women make three times more visits to doctors than do men.

Many of these women are worried about being infected by their nurses and doctors. And many nurses and doctors are concerned about being infected by their patients.

Patti Wetzel, M.D., is a young physician who became fascinated with HIV disease during her medical residency training. She took care of her first AIDS patients in 1987. During her third year of training, she was asked by a local hospital in Fort Worth to head a unit dedicated to caring for AIDS patients. She accepted the job after completing her residency in July 1991.

In September of that year, Dr. Wetzel was drawing blood on a patient with AIDS — a routine procedure. She was accidentally stuck by the needle she had used. Dr. Wetzel made national news in March 1992, when she announced that she had tested positive for HIV antibodies.

Dr. Wetzel is one of only a very few healthcare workers believed to have acquired HIV from an accidental exposure to a needle used on an HIV-infected patient.

"Pretty much everyone I worked with has had a needle stick. They all told me not to worry, minimizing my concerns and fears at the time," she recalled. She had the classic symptoms of an HIV infection about two weeks later — a fever, headache and generally did not feel well. She was vacationing with her husband, an emergency room physician, and when he came down with a cold, she tried to tell herself that she, too, only had a cold.

Her first ELISA test, done soon after the incident, came back with seemingly good news — negative for HIV antibodies. "That made me feel better, even though I knew it was really too soon to be sure because of the window period." In the meantime, she developed a corneal ulcer and swollen lymph glands, both of which disappeared by the end of November.

In mid-December, after three months had passed, it was time to get another HIV test. The blood was drawn on Saturday. By Tuesday, her physician gave her the news — she had been infected.

"The next two weeks, which were over the Christmas holidays, we are really very fuzzy," Dr. Wetzel said. "I don't remember much of those days at all. Basically it was just my husband and myself trying to deal with this news.

"I returned to work in January, and I tried to carry on. It still doesn't seem very real. I'm fine. I'm healthy. I feel fine. I still think a lot of the time this just can't really be. Sometimes I go to my own private lab file to see my lab results. I think this must be a dream, a bad joke. I'm certain that's what many others must feel like."

Dr. Wetzel decided to return to work, caring for people who had developed the diseases associated with HIV, which meant dealing with death and dying every day. Finally she couldn't take the strain any longer.

"The straw that broke the back for me was a female patient," she remembers. "This woman had been infected in 1985 by a blood transfusion given prior to screening. She had been working as a waitress and when she left the restaurant late at night, she was struck with a bullet meant for someone else. She had required surgery and a blood transfusion. A year and a half later, she found out she was HIV infected.

"I had become very close to her, and I really admired her because she had such a positive attitude," Dr. Wetzel said. "Her goal had been to live at least until July because she wanted to see her child graduate from high school in May and head out on her own. In February, she became very ill. She never made it out of the hospital, and she died in early March."

Her patient's death affected Dr. Wetzel profoundly.

Now she is dedicating her life to teach women to understand what they can do to protect themselves from getting HIV, both in the healthcare setting and in their daily lives.

"Since I announced that I was HIV infected, I've had women from across the country call to say that they were infected as well, and they didn't know who to talk to," Dr. Wetzel said. In her years of caring for HIV-infected patients, she's noticed a change in the infected population.

"When I was in medical school, we were almost exclusively seeing a gay male population," she explained. "During my residency, every once in a while we would see an HIV-infected woman. By the time I took this job, out of 700 patients, 70 were women." The hospital even began setting aside a "woman's day" for the women who were uncomfortable coming to the clinic alongside men. While most of the women had been infected as a result of IV drug use, an increasing number of women now coming for care are those whose husbands or sex partners have infected them.

Should People Be Afraid Of Their Caregiver?

Some people panic at the thought of being cared for by an HIV-infected nurse or doctor.

"When the news came out (about her HIV infection), we had one father come in and demand to be tested," Dr. Wetzel said. "He had brought his son in and I had put his son's broken arm in a splint. I never touched the father and yet, because he had been in the same room with me, he was afraid I had given him AIDS."

There is no way that by simply being in the room with Dr. Wetzel, the man could have been infected.

After all the publicity about Kimberly Bergalis, a 23-year-old Florida woman who died of AIDS, and four other people who became HIV infected apparently after being treated by the same dentist, I'm often asked about the safety of healthcare. There are two questions to ask:

1. What is the risk of transmission from the healthcare worker to the patient?
2. How can this risk be reduced?

The case of the Florida dentist is puzzling. Extensive investigation showed that five patients of this AIDS-infected dentist tested positive for HIV antibodies. The evidence strongly suggests that somehow the virus was transmitted by the dentist while he was providing dental care. This incident has been closely studied by public health officials, and to this day they don't know exactly how this occurred. Inadequate cleaning of dental equipment is the likely cause. They do know that the dental office ignored well-established standards for cleaning and sterilizing instruments. To date, this is the only documented case of HIV infection being spread by a healthcare worker.

The idea of being infected by your doctor, nurse or dentist is frightening, but the chances are very small. Tests of more than 15,000 people treated by HIV-infected healthcare workers have found no new cases in which patients were infected as a result.

Many patients don't realize that in order to be infected by a caregiver that caregiver would have to somehow get their own blood into the patient's blood or have sex with the patient.

"In reality, for healthcare workers to pass on an infection to a patient, they would literally have to bleed into the patient, and that's not an easy thing to accomplish," said Barbara Russell, R.N., MPH, CIC, director of infection control for Baptist Hospital of Miami. Ms. Russell has been chairwoman of the HIV Resource Task Force for the American Nurses Association and has also chaired the Florida Nurses Association HIV Task Force. She has testified frequently at Congressional hearings concerning HIV and healthcare workers and has been recognized nationally for her efforts to educate all people about the dangers of HIV disease.

Because surgery involves blood, people do fear being infected by their surgeon. Let's take a look at the likelihood of being infected by a surgeon:

First, the surgeon would need to be infected. A rough estimate is that between 1.5 and 7 per 1,000 surgeons nationwide are infected.

Second, the surgeon would have to be cut during that surgical procedure. Then, the HIV infection would have to be passed on from the surgeon to the patient. For example, the object causing the injury and contaminated with the surgeon's blood would have to contact the patient's wound. The odds of this happening are only 3 in every 1,000 exposures.

The odds are small, but not zero.

In order to reduce these risks even further, the CDC, the American Medical Association and other healthcare organizations are encouraging testing of any healthcare provider who performs certain procedures in which the patient is more likely to come into contact with the blood of the provider. If the healthcare worker is positive, he or she is encouraged to advise patients before the procedure, or to voluntarily abstain from doing a procedure.

Because this virus is not spread easily, most physicians, nurses and other healthcare workers can continue to safely provide care even if they are infected.

"Physicians and healthcare providers don't want to put their patients at risk any more than they themselves want to be at risk," said Dr. Wetzel.

Should Caregivers Be Afraid Of Their Patients?

The truth is, the healthcare provider is at far greater risk of being infected by a patient than the patient is of being infected by the caregiver.

Dr. Wetzel's story illustrates why healthcare workers are afraid — afraid to take care of infected patients and of being tested for HIV. Being stuck by a needle that was used on a patient is every healthcare worker's nightmare.

As one nurse said, "I've been accidentally stuck by used needles, but I refuse to have the test done because I'm scared to death of what I'll find. What if I find out I'm HIV infected? I have two children to bring up and support. What if I lose my job and my health insurance?"

Healthcare workers have been closely monitored since 1983, and, to date, 29 providers have been documented by the CDC as being infected as a result of having cared for an HIV-infected patient. Three have AIDS.

Another 18 say they were exposed on the job but that hasn't been proven. Sixty-six infected healthcare workers have no other known risk factors and may have been infected on the job. Eleven other cases from outside of the United States have been reported to the CDC. The majority of these providers were infected as a result of having been accidentally stuck by a needle used on a person with HIV. It is estimated that after a significant needle stick injury from an infected patient, the odds of becoming infected are about 1 in 250.

The true number of healthcare workers infected by HIV is obviously not known, since not every healthcare worker is tested after a needle stick injury, and not every injury is reported to the CDC. However, hepatitis B is a much larger problem for healthcare workers. As many as 300 healthcare workers die each year as a result of hepatitis B they acquired on the job. There is, however, a vaccine against hepatitis B available to all healthcare workers.

It must be remembered that healthcare workers can become infected in the same way as anyone else — through sexual intercourse.

What About Outside The Hospital?

Standards of infection control are extremely strict and closely monitored in the hospital setting, but may not be as strict in your doctor's or dentist's office. You should feel free to question your healthcare provider about what steps are being taken to protect you from infection.

If your healthcare provider does not want or isn't able to answer your questions or concerns, perhaps you should find another provider who understands your right to be informed. Most of the healthcare professionals I work with understand their patients' need to know what's being done to protect them.

Some questions to ask are:

• Does he or she wash hands between patients?
• Does he or she change gloves between patients?

- Are disposable needles used to draw blood?
- What happens to the needle after it's used?
- How are the instruments cleaned or sterilized?

Please understand that not all instruments used need to be sterilized. However, items that penetrate the body, coming into contact with blood and other body fluids, must be sterilized before being used again. Instruments that simply touch intact skin should be cleaned with a disinfectant. If you ever take part in a health screening in which your cholesterol or blood sugar levels are checked with just a small prick of the finger for a blood sample, make sure the provider changes his or her gloves for each new person. And make sure the disposable needles used are being discarded after every use. Most of these specialized instruments have a safety device which requires the dirty needle to be discarded before a new one is used. All instruments used should be kept free of blood.

Risky Cosmetic Procedures

A friend of mine was undergoing a facial during which the cosmetologist pricks the skin with a needle to cleanse the clogged pores. My friend asked beforehand if disposable needles, discarded after each use, were being used. She was reassured when shown how the disposable needle system worked.

If you have a deep cleaning facial mask, manicure or pedicure, you should be just as concerned about the cleanliness of the cosmetic devices and the setting as you are about your doctor's or dentist's office. Although the chances of transmitting HIV are very small in these settings, there is a slight risk. All scissors, clippers and the like should be cleaned in a suitable disinfectant, although it's not necessary that they be sterilized.

"The fear of AIDS should not overwhelm or overcome you so that you live in constant fear," said Ms. Russell. "But it has taught us to use some common sense and judgment both when it comes to our personal lives, as well as in the healthcare setting."

We should keep in mind the global HIV epidemic remains largely spread by sexual contact and injection drug use.

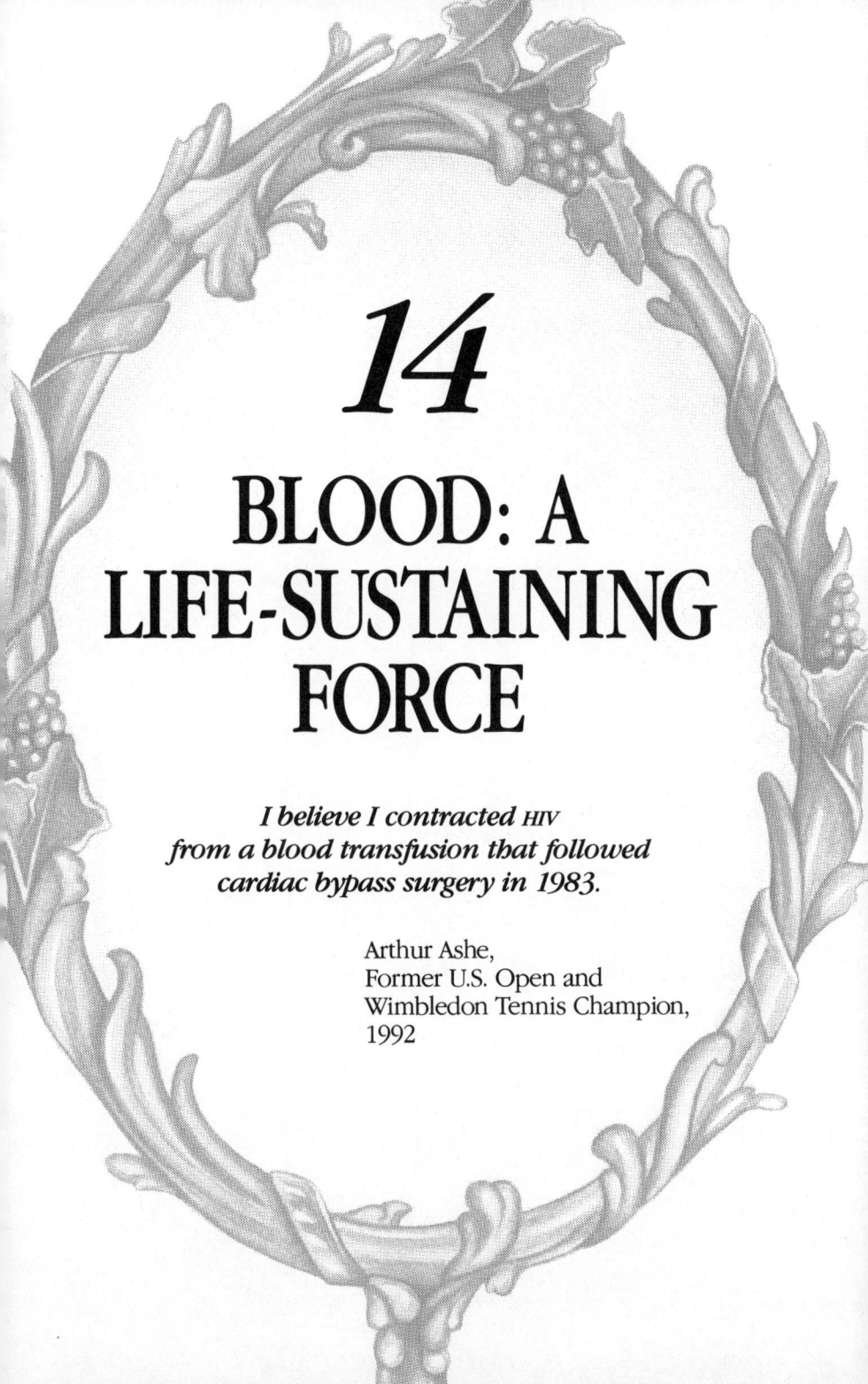

14

BLOOD: A LIFE-SUSTAINING FORCE

I believe I contracted HIV from a blood transfusion that followed cardiac bypass surgery in 1983.

Arthur Ashe,
Former U.S. Open and
Wimbledon Tennis Champion,
1992

*I*t was 1982 when researchers began to suspect that HIV disease might be transmitted by blood. The very blood that sustains our bodies — and, in some critical situations, restores our life — could also be the route of this deadly virus into our bodies.

By 1984, 18 cases of AIDS — 8 of them in women — had been linked to blood transfusions. The idea that blood brought death instead of life was awful to contemplate. Blood became a highly charged subject when linked with AIDS.

It wasn't until March 1985, that the first test, the ELISA (Enzyme Linked Immunosorbant Assay), was licensed by the Food and Drug Administration for routine screening of the blood supply. Protection of our blood supply has been one of the highest public health priorities.

Comparing the number of people infected through blood before and after 1985 shows how effective measures to protect the nation's blood supply have been: From 1981 until testing began in 1985, 4,519 adults and 294 children were identified as contracting AIDS from blood. Since 1985, only 18 adults and 2 children have been identified as having AIDS as a result of a transfusion. It must be noted, however, that there is no way of knowing how many people are HIV infected who have not yet developed AIDS or who have not been reported to the CDC.

The risk today of acquiring HIV from blood and blood products is minimal. The average national risk is between 1 in 40,000 and 1 in 250,000 per unit of blood given. That's compared to the risk of death from pregnancy of 1 in 4,250; smoking 20 cigarettes a day, 1 in 100; of dying in a car accident, 1 in 5,900; or dying of the flu, 1 in 5,000.

Even given the dramatic improvement in the purity of the blood supply, people tend to be more afraid of having a blood transfusion than of having unprotected sex or sharing a dirty needle — behaviors that are much more risky.

Can I *Give* Blood Without Fear Of Being Infected?

In fact, people early on in the epidemic began to stay away from blood drives, fearing they could get this disease by *donating* blood, as well as from receiving a blood transfusion. "Out of 13 million donations of blood per year," said Bruce Lenes, M.D., medical director of the American Red Cross, South Florida Region, "we believe there has not been one single instance of HIV infection related to the donation of blood." Every unit of blood is drawn with a new sterile needle, and all equipment used is sterile, so it's impossible to become infected when donating.

If you feel healthy and meet all donor eligibility criteria (that is, if you are not a carrier of HIV or other infectious diseases transmitted through blood, such as hepatitis), then please donate blood when asked. Giving blood to save the lives of others is an important public service.

Blood Transfusions:
Should You Be Afraid?

Should you be afraid to receive a blood transfusion if your doctor suggests it?

"The bottom line is that a person should be given blood only when the benefits of that transfusion outweigh the risk," said Dr. Lenes. "We cannot make blood transfusions 100 percent safe, even with today's science and medicine. The decision about whether or not to receive a blood transfusion is an individual one. Physician and patient must look at individual patient circumstances at a given time. Ninety-nine percent of individuals will benefit from receiving the blood. It's only that fraction of one percent with a bad result, and that is the person we're concerned about."

Tennis great Arthur Ashe had open heart surgery in 1983 (before HIV testing was available). The surgery and blood transfusion gave him years of life. But the blood was infected with HIV and Ashe contracted AIDS.

It was in 1983 that Miamian Doug Segal received a letter advising him that the blood product he used as a hemophiliac was tainted, composed of blood donated by a man with AIDS. (Hemophiliacs use a product made from blood. Prior to testing for AIDS and a change in the manufacture of the blood product so that the HIV virus was destroyed, there were 1,812 adult and 173 child hemophiliacs known to be infected by blood products. Since 1985, none have been identified.) Segal died in 1988, leaving behind his wife, Ellen, and three young children.

Today there are. many safeguards in place to protect people from an infected unit of blood, but, as with any medical procedure, there remains a minimal risk.

Blood Donation

Today's blood supply is based on a volunteer system of donation that is closely monitored and tested. Every unit of blood is tested for HIV, as well as for many other diseases, including hepatitis B and C.

In fact, blood is tested for two types of HIV — HIV1, the viral strain most commonly found in the United States, and HIV2, a form that is found predominantly in Africa and other parts of the world, with only a few cases reported in the United States.

Every person volunteering to donate a unit of blood is asked a series of direct questions to find out if that individual may be at risk for HIV infection. If there is any indication that an individual may be at risk, he or she is not allowed to give blood.

Questions include:

- Have you ever had sex with an IV drug user or someone who is HIV infected?
- Have you ever received drugs or money for sex?
- Have you had sex with another man (if you're a male donor)?
- Have you had sex with a prostitute in the last year?
- Do you have any sexually transmitted disease(s)?

There are other reasons, besides AIDS exposure, for being excluded from donating blood. These include: malaria or visiting an area where there is malaria; having had hepatitis; or travel outside of the United States within the last three years to certain countries.

Knowing that some people may not answer all questions truthfully, another step has been devised by blood collection facilities to help people "save face." After the initial questionnaire has been completed, donors have the option of placing one of two computerized bar code labels on their forms. One code stands for "Use my blood," the other for "Don't use my blood." Only the blood bank staff knows which label is selected, and the blood with the "Don't use" code is discarded.

Every unit of donated blood is then tested for hepatitis, syphilis, HIV1, HIV2 and several other diseases.

Individuals who test positive for these infections are notified of their results. However, blood bank officials are quick to point out that people wishing to know their test results should *not* use the blood center as a testing site. Using a blood center in this manner may put people who receive blood at risk. People who want to know their HIV status should talk with their own physician or go to a public health clinic for testing.

A detailed and highly confidential recordkeeping system automatically tracks ineligible blood donors and prevents donations from such donors with prior positive tests.

If a blood center finds that a donor whose previously donated blood tested negative is now positive for HIV, a program called "look back" is initiated. This system of looking back on previous recipients of blood donations is necessary because a person could have donated blood during the "window period," when infected blood might test negative. The blood bank will contact the hospital where the first donated blood was sent. The hospital will then attempt to trace the patient who received that blood, and will alert the physician to what has happened. The doctor can then call the patient and offer counseling and testing to see if he or she is infected with HIV.

Why Isn't All Donated Blood Safe?

With all of the safeguards, why isn't the blood supply 100 percent free óf HIV? The first reason is the window period — those six months when a person's blood may test negative for the HIV antibodies, yet still be infectious. That's why it's important not to give blood if you have recently participated in risk behaviors.

People often ask why donated blood can't be stored for six months and retested to check for HIV disease. That's because once the blood is outside the body, it cannot manufacture the antibodies which show up in HIV screening. If the blood tests negative for HIV at the time of donation, then it will also test negative again after six months of storage.

Sometimes it's tough to say no to blood donation: for example, if your employer is urging employees to give to a local blood drive, or if a family member or close friend asks as a personal favor to give blood for someone in a critical medical condition.

But if you have reason to think you may be at risk for HIV, it is okay to say no to those asking or tell the blood bank staff that you are not eligible to donate. In some states it is a felony to give blood if you think or know you are infected with HIV. While I don't condone lying, it is better to refuse in a way that is comfortable for you than to give possibly contaminated blood to someone. I have known people who refused, saying they had "had hepatitis," or that they "pass out at the sight of needles."

Since the onset of the AIDS epidemic, physicians themselves have become more reluctant to use transfusions. In the past, we used to "top up" people. If they were a little anemic, we'd give them blood to make them feel better more quickly. The criteria for giving a blood transfusion was less strict. Today physicians recommend that unless patients' hemoglobin is critically low, they're better off waiting for the body's natural reproduction of blood, even if it means feeling slightly weak for a while. The bottom line is that fewer transfusions are being given.

If your doctor thinks you need a blood transfusion, ask what the risks are if you do not have a transfusion. You and your doctor, together, should weigh those risks against the small risk of getting an infection from blood.

Approximately 100 to 200 units of HIV-infected blood will be given in the United States per year, despite the elaborate screening and testing process. People who receive infected blood will most likely become infected and will spread HIV to others.

Because blood transfusions are used more sparingly today — primarily in life or death situations — it's important to know that one-half of the people receiving infected blood die before they leave the hospital because of the illness or injury itself. Of those who leave the hospital, another one-half will die from that injury or illness before they die of HIV disease.

Remember, the chances of getting AIDS from a blood transfusion are much smaller than your chances of being in a car accident on your way to the hospital.

What If I Don't Want To Use The Community's Blood Supply?

There are times when blood is absolutely necessary to sustain life. Consider the occurrence of a major injury, when one is in danger of bleeding to death without additional blood. Or major surgery, when substantial blood loss is anticipated. In these cases, the minuscule risk of getting HIV-infected blood should not deter one from obtaining a life-saving transfusion.

Sometimes, however, you can plan ahead by saving your own blood. This is known as autologous blood transfusion. You can donate blood ahead of time or have your doctor collect it during the operation or both.

1. Donating your own blood before surgery

If your doctor thinks you'll need blood during surgery, and you have a few weeks before the surgery is scheduled, then autologous blood donation may be an option. You will be directed to a facility where your blood will be taken, and your doctor will write a medical order noting how many units of blood you will need.

Usually a blood center will collect only one unit of blood a week, so it is best to start the process at least four to six weeks prior to surgery. You may be asked to take special iron pills each day to supplement iron in your blood. Each donation of blood will take from one to two hours of your time, and you may be billed for this service.

Your blood will then be stored until you need it, or if you don't need it, it will be released for others to use. Because of the limited life of stored blood, it won't be kept forever. Storing your own blood is only practical if you have a planned operation, are sufficiently healthy and can afford to do so.

As for having your blood collected and kept frozen by one of the commercial blood storage centers popping up around the country, keep in mind that very rarely can that blood get to you in a true emergency. Most likely, you'll need that blood immediately, before the commercial bank has a chance to prepare the blood and deliver it for transfusion. It is often impractical to get that blood at the time of an emergency because you are in a place far away from the storage site, or you are not in good enough condition to tell anyone where your blood is stored.

2. Collecting blood during surgery

Blood salvage is a procedure which allows blood to be collected during surgery, processed and then given back to you if needed.

This option is not open to everyone. For example, if you have an infection, you won't be given your own blood. Or if there's not enough time to collect the blood your doctor thinks you will need, you may have to rely on the community's supply.

Some pregnant women, concerned that they may need surgery and perhaps blood during childbirth, opt to give their own blood in advance. While this may eliminate some fears of a pregnant woman, she should be aware that the overwhelming majority of women do not need blood at birth. And while it is believed there is minimal risk to the fetus if the mother chooses to give blood, there are still some unknowns concerning the effects of donating blood during pregnancy. (If a physician suggests that a mother-to-be opt for autologous blood donation, it's generally because the physician is more concerned about the woman's emotional state than her chances for acquiring HIV or other diseases.)

Can I Ask A Friend Or Relative To Donate Blood For Me?

Some people believe that asking close friends or family members to donate blood for a loved one is a good protection against infected blood. While this may seem logical, it's not necessarily true. Family members may not be honest about their risk behaviors and may not be the "safest" donors around. Asking people close to you to donate blood may put them in the position of having to say yes, when they know their blood may not be safe. It is generally believed that the volunteer blood supply is at least as safe as blood donated by friends and relatives.

I once had a patient who asked her boyfriend to donate blood for her. I knew her boyfriend had some homosexual experiences, making him a risky donor, but the woman did not know of his past. In this case, the woman was better off getting blood from an anonymous donor through the general blood supply.

Should I Be Tested If I've Had A Blood Transfusion?

When Arthur Ashe announced that he had AIDS as a result of a blood transfusion, many people who had also had blood transfusions panicked. Telephone hot lines at blood banks nationwide were ringing off the hook.

If you are concerned that you may have been infected because you received a blood transfusion, then please consider getting tested. If you received the blood more than six months ago, and you now test negative for HIV, then you can put your fears to rest — unless you've engaged in some other risky behavior since then.

I think anyone who had a transfusion before 1985 (before blood was screened for HIV), or who had sex with someone receiving a blood transfusion before 1985, should be tested.

Remember Joyce, whose husband had a transfusion in 1984. He had been concerned about possible infection all of these years, but did not get tested until 1991, after a bout with shingles — a fairly common condition, but more common among HIV-infected individuals. He tested positive. So did Joyce. Based on other tests, it appears her infection was fairly recent. If her husband had been tested earlier, precautions might have been taken, and Joyce might not have become infected.

Is Blood Safe Elsewhere In The World?

We have adopted a philosophy of testing blood in the United States, but that's not the case in all other countries. In Romania in May 1990, officials reported that 617 children had been diagnosed with AIDS, whereas the total number of recorded AIDS cases in Romania was then only 670. Most of the children were living in institutions so that few of the mothers were found and tested. Only five percent of the mothers were HIV infected, ruling out mother to child as the primary route of infection for these children.

Contaminated blood was found to be the primary source of infection. In Romania, it was common medical practice to give small amounts of blood to children who were undernourished, as most of these youngsters were. Also this country had little access to sterilized needles and equipment, so a second route of infection was indicated. In addition, the blood supply was not being screened for HIV. After this report, the Romanian Ministry of

Health began testing all institutionalized children under three years of age. Of more than 10,500 tested by June 1990, 10 percent were HIV infected.

According to Lyle Petersen, M.D., Chief of the Population Study Section, Division of HIV/AIDS for the Centers for Disease Control, "There is no systematic study on who is screening blood and who is not." In most developed countries, such as the European nations, "the blood supply is as safe there as it is here," he said. All blood is also screened in Japan.

In most Latin American countries, blood is screened in major cities, but there is no guarantee in remote areas of these countries. If you go to Africa, for the most part, all bets are off for getting a safe transfusion, since there is a high population of HIV-infected people, and the blood supply in most areas is not screened for infection. In sub-Saharan Africa, 10 percent of AIDS cases by 1990 were the result of transfusions with infected blood. In Asia, it depends on the country.

"When traveling abroad, the general rule would be to avoid blood transfusions if you possibly can, particularly in Third World countries," Dr. Petersen said. Again, weigh the risk of not having a transfusion with the risk of having one, taking into consideration whether or not the area's blood bank screens for HIV and other diseases.

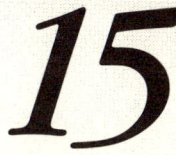

15

MYTHS, QUESTIONS AND ANSWERS ABOUT AIDS

The best protection against the AIDS virus right now, barring abstinence, is the use of a condom. A condom should be used during sexual relations from start to finish with everyone whom you are not absolutely sure is free of the AIDS virus.

C. Everett Koop, M.D.,
Former Surgeon General
of the United States

*T*rue statement: Anybody can get AIDS, but nobody has to.

You may think that you're well informed about AIDS, and by the time you've read this far you probably are. And you may have seen AIDS reports on television and radio, and information printed in newspapers and books. But even well-informed, intelligent people have misconceptions. Here are some of the most frequently asked — as well as unusual — questions about AIDS.

Q. Why do we know so little about AIDS?

A. So many people tell me that the scariest thing about AIDS is that we know so little about it. True, we don't know as much as we'd like because if we did, we could stop this epidemic. But we do know some important things:

- What causes AIDS.
- How it is spread.
- How to protect ourselves from it.
- How to test for it.

What we don't know is how to cure it. We also don't know why some people get infected after having sex only once with an infected person, while others can have sex with an infected person many times before becoming infected; and we don't know why some people die within a few months of infection and others live for many years.

Q. Do only gay men get AIDS?

A. As long as women believe this myth, they and their children will continue to die of AIDS in ever-increasing numbers. The World Health Organization estimates that, during the 1990s, more than three million women and children will die from HIV infection. In New York City, AIDS is already the leading cause of death among women between the ages of 25 and 35. Nationwide, AIDS is the fifth leading cause of death in women of childbearing age. So don't think that AIDS can't happen to you.

Q. Are gay women safe from AIDS?

A. Gay women have been deeply affected by this epidemic. Many feel a responsibility to work in AIDS projects and have been involved in taking care of people with AIDS. They have also been affected because of the increased homophobia which the AIDS epidemic has prompted. Although gay women are at the lowest risk group for getting AIDS, lesbians are not immune to the disease.

Some gay women have sex with men, often with gay or bisexual men. Or in trying to become pregnant, they may have sex with men who are at high risk. Some women may have used semen for artificial insemination from a donor who is infected with HIV. Like other members of the general population, some gay women may be IV drug abusers and at risk for acquiring the virus from needle sharing.

It is thought that the AIDS virus can be transmitted by oral sex. This means a gay woman might pass on the virus to a partner through oral sex. It is also conceivable, but not documented, that sharing sex devices like vibrators or dildos could be a means of transmission. Gay women should practice safer sex. If they perform oral sex on each other, they should be careful that a rubber dam, a square of rubber latex or a piece of non-micro-wavable plastic wrap be doubled over and placed over the genital areas of the woman on whom oral sex is to be performed.

Q. Will a cure soon be found?

A. Don't rely on great advances in research to find a cure for this virus anytime soon. Some people say, "I'm not going to worry about getting the virus, because they'll find a cure for it before I get full-blown AIDS." This is probably not true. Although we know a lot more now about how to control the virus, it's a very difficult disease to cure, and no cure or vaccine is on the horizon. It is true that we know how to prevent and manage some of the infections that AIDS patients are prone to, but at present AIDS is still a 100 percent fatal disease.

Q. Can I get AIDS from a mosquito bite?

A. No. Mosquitoes and other insects don't spread HIV. For one thing, the amount of blood a mosquito takes from a human is not enough to spread the virus. The AIDS virus does not survive in the mosquito and it is not transmitted through the salivary glands of the mosquito like other diseases such as malaria. Think about it: If insect bites could spread the virus, there would be many more cases among older people, children and people who are not having sex, but are bitten by mosquitos.

Q. Should I avoid using public bathrooms, telephones or eating utensils which infected people may have used?

A. No. Not one of the tens of thousands of household members in homes shared with an infected person have tested positive unless they've had sex or shared needles with that person. AIDS is spread through exchange of body fluids such as semen and blood.

Q. Can I get AIDS by donating blood?

A. No. Every unit of blood collected from donors is drawn with a sterile disposable needle and goes into a sterile bag. It's impossible to get AIDS from donating blood.

Q. Can I get AIDS by being in the same room as an infected person, or by hugging or shaking the person's hand?

A. No. People have the mistaken notion that HIV is like other viruses such as chicken pox or flu, which are easy to catch from others. If this were true, almost everybody would be infected within a very short period of time and that's not the case. AIDS is a difficult disease to get except from sex and blood.

Q. Can I get AIDS if I use birth control prevention?

A. Unless you use condoms, you are at risk of contracting AIDS. Birth control devices may protect against pregnancy, but not against HIV infection or sexually transmitted diseases. If you are using some form of birth control — including the pill, diaphragm, sponge, IUD — you also need to use a condom. Remember, just as a birth control pill won't stop you from getting mumps, it won't stop you from getting the AIDS virus or other sexually transmitted diseases either.

Q. If I have a hysterectomy or have my tubes tied, can I still get AIDS?

A. Most assuredly you are still at risk. These procedures make you unable to conceive, but you can still be infected by HIV.

Q. I've heard that your digestive juices kill the virus if you swallow semen. Isn't oral sex safe?

A. Don't risk your life on the basis of this old myth. Early in the epidemic we thought that HIV was killed or inactivated by digestive juices. Now we have seen many cases of AIDS which began with oral sex. Even if the virus were inactivated in the stomach, it still has to pass through the mouth, where infection can readily take place.

Q. Where do I get dental dams and non-microwaveable plastic wrap?

A. Dental dams are hard to get. You have to order them through dental supply stores. Plastic wrap is available in supermarkets. Be sure you get the non-microwaveable kind.

Q. Don't I need to prick a hole in the tip of the condom so the sperm will have a place to go?

A. Definitely not true. Your partner's testicles will not blow up if the condom is sealed. This is a myth. Please, never put a hole in a condom you are about to use for sex.

Q. If I use a spermicide with nonoxynol-9, do I have to use a condom also?

A. While nonoxynol-9 will inactivate the virus in a test tube, no studies have been conducted to prove that this is true in the vagina. Please don't rely on the spermicide alone; use it with a condom.

Q. If my partner is HIV positive, but doesn't have AIDS, can he infect me?

A. He can. Being HIV positive means he carries the virus, has the antibodies to the virus and can transmit the virus to others. Anyone who is HIV positive is infectious, even though he or she may not have symptoms of disease.

Q. If I've been to my doctor and had a complete physical exam and blood tests, has he or she automatically tested me for AIDS as well?

A. Unless your doctor asked your permission to do an AIDS test on you and you have given your consent or you have specifically asked for the test to be done, the test won't be done. Don't assume a clean bill of health means you're not infected unless you've had the AIDS test. And remember, the test must be specifically ordered.

Myths: Sex And Love

There are a lot of myths about sex and love. Here are a few:

"I love you and I would never give you AIDS."

This virus knows nothing about feelings people have for each other. If a man loves you, he wouldn't intentionally transmit AIDS to you, but this virus has a mind of its own. If your partner is infected, it doesn't matter whether he loves you, he can still infect you.

"I can tell by looking at someone if he shoots drugs or is bisexual or has AIDS. If I don't have sex with people like him, I won't get AIDS."

Let me shatter this myth about judging by appearances with this true story.

As a physician, I have a special interest in AIDS, but I also have a regular family practice. Michael is a prominent married lawyer. He came to see me because of a fever he'd had for a week. I tried to find out why but couldn't find a reason for his chills and headache. I admitted him to the hospital for additional tests. My associate, who at that time had an almost exclusive interest in AIDS patients, was on vacation.

When he returned, I discussed Michael's condition with him. He asked if I had given Michael an HIV test. I hadn't tested Michael because I didn't believe HIV was his problem. And, in any case, he was married with children. I told my colleague, "You have to realize there are other diseases out there besides HIV." Fortunately my colleague was wise enough to remind me that even married men get AIDS. Michael's AIDS test came back positive. It turned out he was bisexual and HIV infected, even though he was married.

I have seen hundreds of HIV-infected patients. I know more than I sometimes care to about this disease. And even I was fooled by appearances. You cannot know if people are at high risk, or if they carry this virus, unless you ask them and unless they have been tested.

"Attractive, well-groomed, intelligent and nice people don't get AIDS."

Most of my AIDS patients look like the girl or guy next door. And most are beautiful, athletic, well-groomed, intelligent and likable people, exactly the sort of people you'd probably like to know.

"Love and intercourse go hand in hand."

Real, lasting love is about caring, trusting, respect and friendship, not about sex.

"I have to have sex by the time I'm out of high school, otherwise I'm missing out."

The truth is, people enjoy sex well into their 80s, so there's really no need to rush into having sex before you're ready. Most of the teens I know may be physically, but not psychologically, ready for sex.

"Everyone is doing it, so I have to, too."

No, you don't. In reality, there are millions of teenagers and adults who have chosen not to have sex.

"Once I've had sex, I can't become celibate."

In truth, once people have become sexually active, they often remain sexually active. However, there are many people who, having had sexual relationships in the past, have realized that either the timing is not right for them, or their relationship isn't right for sex. They choose to abstain from sex. Sometimes these people call themselves "born-again virgins."

"The only way to avoid getting AIDS is to give up all sex, unless I'm in a long-term, monogamous relationship."

This is really two myths in one. You can be in a long-term, monogamous relationship with somebody who's HIV infected. And so monogamy is not necessarily a barrier to the AIDS virus. The other myth is that you have to give up all sex. This depends on your definition of sex. If holding hands and hugging are included in your definition of sex, you don't have to give up all sex. Giving up sexual intercourse will definitely help prevent your getting AIDS.

"A single exposure is not dangerous. I have nothing to worry about unless I've had multiple sexual partners."

Don't fool yourself. A single sexual encounter is like playing Russian Roulette.

"Masturbation is bad for me."

Masturbation is a normal human behavior and contrary to popular belief, masturbation will not cause blindness, make your clitoris fall off or put hair on your hands. I know. I'm a doctor, and I've examined many people who masturbate. Remember, masturbation has never been known to cause pregnancy or sexually transmitted diseases.

I spend so much time thinking and talking about this epidemic, that sometimes I assume everybody understands as much as I do. But people understand this disease only in terms of their own life experiences or interpret what I'm saying much differently than I intended. This is how myths are created and perpetuated.

My own son taught me this years ago. By the time he was 10 years old, he'd heard me constantly talk about the horrors of the new epidemic. One day he asked me, "Mom, why wouldn't you want to give this virus to somebody else?" I tried to explain, again, the horrors of this disease. He rephrased the question, "So why wouldn't you want to give it to anyone else?"

I began to suspect that my child was a monster, until he asked another question. "If you give this to somebody, doesn't it mean you won't have AIDS anymore?"

Unfortunately, once you have AIDS, you can't give it away.

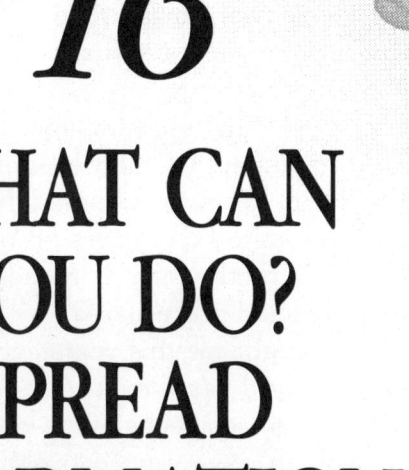

16

WHAT CAN YOU DO? SPREAD INFORMATION, NOT AIDS

Now is the time for global solidarity against a common enemy. Now is the time for us to share our knowledge.

Elizabeth Taylor

*I*n 1989 I met a physician who worked for the gold mines in Johannesburg, South Africa. Most of the miners came from the homelands, lived in barracks and didn't visit their families for a year at a time.

A few prostitutes served the men in the barracks and there was a growing problem of AIDS. I asked the doctor how he was treating his patients, and he replied, "As soon as they are diagnosed with AIDS, they're sent back to their homeland."

I then asked how he was educating the miners about this disease to keep them from spreading it and was horrified when he said, "Dr. Sack, I'm a doctor. Education is none of my business!"

In shock, I asked, "If it isn't your business, then whose is it?"

"I don't know," he replied.

In the three months it took to write this book, 7,000 people in America have died of AIDS. That's three to four people every hour. World-wide, 30 people every hour are diagnosed with HIV disease.

Globally, treatment remains too expensive for people who need it. The total budget for the average national AIDS program in the developing world in 1990 was less than the cost for caring for just 15 people with AIDS in the United States.

In the United States the cost of caring for all people with HIV infection in 1991 was estimated to be $5.8 billion and is expected to rise by 21 percent by 1994.

While the scientific community is doing everything possible to find a way to stop this epidemic, there is no cure on the horizon. It's unrealistic to expect a vaccine to protect us from being infected with HIV anytime soon.

Our only inoculation against this disease is getting rid of the ignorance, shame and denial that surround AIDS, and to realize that AIDS is everyone's responsibility.

The AIDS epidemic is unlike any other epidemic this world has ever experienced. It forces us as a society to delve into areas we'd prefer to keep under cover, issues such as sexual preference, promiscuity, extramarital affairs, prostitution, poverty, drug addiction, domestic violence and child abuse.

To stop the spread of this disease and save lives, many of us will have to overcome our embarrassment or confront our personal beliefs about moral issues.

I am convinced that the only way we'll end this epidemic is if each person believes it is his or her responsibility to teach others. It starts first with the individual making needed changes in his or her sexual practices. Then each person has the responsibility for teaching another, so that whole communities of people will have the information they need to stop this disease.

This includes mothers teaching their children and their friends; doctors and nurses educating patients; the entertainment industry stopping glamorization of casual, unprotected sex; the pornographic industry finding ways to photograph or write about sexual escapades that include a condom and other safer sex practices.

In 1987 during a trip to South Africa I tried to reach the black community. To do this, I planned to meet with witch doctors who are entrusted with the care of their tribes.

It's not easy to get an interview with a witch doctor . . . you can't just pick up the phone and call one, but I was able to get an influential black man to take me into a township near Durban. We went to the shack belonging to the witch doctor. He came out to greet us, dressed in his native garb and rattling some herbs in his hand. He invited me to eat some of these herbs.

This tiny, wizened old man looked me up and down, and seemed pleased that a white doctor from America wanted to talk with him. I asked if he had heard about AIDS, and he replied that he had.

He said he was not really concerned about this new disease because although he understood it was going to affect many of his people, he knew how to cure them. He had a potion in mind, mixing some herbs and bark together.

In a comforting voice, he told me I really shouldn't worry about AIDS because the disease was easily cured.

For a brief moment, I believed in his magical smile and charismatic manner and his promises of a cure. Unfortunately, it didn't take me long to realize how dangerous his comforting promise was.

Because of his power and position, the witch doctor would give false comfort to his people, who would believe him when he offered them a cure instead of a prevention. In effect, he would be reponsible for many, many deaths.

A few days later, I went to Zululand and tried to visit the witch doctor there. For two days, the Zulu people watched to see if I would be granted a meeting with their witch doctor. Just hours before I was to leave, I was told I could meet with him.

This witch doctor was young, handsome, intelligent and worldly. He understood the AIDS epidemic, that it was sexually transmitted, that there was no cure and that condoms were important in preventing the spread of the disease.

However, he said, "It is not my place to tell people to use condoms. I will lose all credibility as a witch doctor if I do."

The tragedy is that Africa has been the continent hardest hit, with 6.5 million reported cases of HIV infection in 1992. *Heterosexual sex is the primary means of infection there, with men and women equally affected.*

I'll never know how many lives I've saved by telling people how to protect themselves from AIDS, but you don't have to be a doctor to save lives.

A South African friend of mine, Brenda Eckstein, who had heard me talk about AIDS, spent some time thinking about what she could to do stop the epidemic in South Africa. As chairman of the Toastmistresses Club in Pietermaritzburg, she invited me to travel from America to my homeland to give the keynote speech on AIDS to about 200 women. The women involved in this club were leaders in their own fields. If each woman could go back to her individual group and teach others, this would be the start of an educational process that was lacking.

These women were teachers who shared their knowledge with other teachers and their students, business owners who later taught their employees and their customers, civic-minded women who volunteered their service wherever it was most needed.

I was also invited to speak to school children, doctors, nurses, the news media, hospice workers and to the lay public during my visit.

Information imparted through this one invitation reached many people who, in turn, became aware of the serious threat of AIDS and were willing to start teaching about it.

Many women have found ways to educate others about AIDS. I've discussed a few in this book: Barbara Russell, R.N., an infection control nurse; Patti Wetzel, M.D., a physician infected with HIV; Ellen Bukstel-Segal, a widow whose husband died from AIDS; and my patients who have bravely gone out to speak to others about their disease.

There are many ways you can make a difference. Here's just a few suggestions on how you can get involved:

Empower yourself with information. Learn all you can about how to protect yourself and those you love from AIDS. And then look for opportunities to share that information. For example, if you are a hairdresser, talk to your clients; if you're a college student, talk to your dorm mates or your sorority sisters; if you're a doctor, talk to your patients.

Believe in your right to protect yourself from possible infection. Learn to say no to unprotected sex or other risky behaviors.

Practice what you preach. Remember the mother who was so concerned about her daughter using condoms that she forgot to use them herself? It's easy to tell others what they should be doing to prevent the spread of AIDS. It's more difficult to realize that you, too, should be doing the same. This goes for grandmothers as well as moms and teens.

"Each one, teach one." That's a slogan I've seen on T-shirts. Whether you're talking to a teenager, a friend, a partner or your parents, don't overlook an opportunity to teach others about preventing HIV disease. If you belong to a church or community organization, call a meeting and invite a local health expert to talk about HIV disease and AIDS. Encourage your friends and family to attend. Support sex education programs in your local schools.

Have a family powwow. If you think your children are old enough to begin understanding what AIDS is and how it can be prevented, have a family meeting. Women often tell me that it's difficult to speak to their children about AIDS, sex and condoms. But if we don't talk to our children about preventing the spread of HIV disease, we may find ourselves talking to them about more difficult issues, such as death, dying and burial plans.

Girls' night out. If you and your friends are uncomfortable or embarrassed to discuss sex or condom use with your partners, get a group together and go visit a condom shop or local drugstore. Together look at the many options available. Buy a few, take them home and practice putting a condom on a banana or cucumber. Practice telling a partner that you won't have sex without a condom and prepare for any of the responses you might get. There may be a lot of giggling and laughing going on during this girls' night out, and that will help you discharge your embarrassment. Keep working through the laughter until you can talk about condoms with no awkwardness at all.

Speak out about the need to assure that adequate medical care is available for everyone, no matter what their economic background. This is an issue that goes beyond HIV disease. Until we as a nation address the inequity of healthcare services, we won't be able to assure that people receive the care needed to stay healthy. Women are particularly affected by the lack of healthcare services since they are less likely to have health insurance. And often they are the sole provider for their families. Until the Centers for Disease Control definition of AIDS is changed to include the HIV infections women are prone to, many will not be identified as having AIDS. This means women will not have access to the Social Security disability benefits to which they may be entitled.

Reach out with compassion to those who are coping with HIV disease. Whether it's a friend who is infected, or a co-worker who is caring for a loved one who has AIDS, show your understanding and support in whatever way possible. Fight the disease, not the people with it.

If you are HIV infected, consider sharing your story with others.
You could have a tremendous impact on people who would
prefer to deny the existence of this disease and their vul-
nerability to infection.

Sometimes I have moments when I feel defeated. How
can we end this epidemic? But on balance I feel hopeful
about the ending HIV disease when I see women support-
ing one another in taking back power over our own bodies
and lives, in getting information out, in breaking through
the myths into compassion.

John Donne expressed my sentiments and hopes well
when he wrote *For Whom The Bell Tolls* in 1624:

> No man is an island, entire of itself; every man is a piece
> of the continent, a part of the main; if a clod be washed
> away by the sea, Europe is the less, as well as if a prom-
> ontory were, as well as if a manor of thy friends or of
> thine own were; any man's death diminishes me, because
> I am involved in mankind; and therefore never send to
> know for whom the bell tolls; it tolls for thee.

What will this epidemic do to this world? To our
children? I often wonder. I think a lot about AIDS and my
role in this epidemic. I have been intellectually and emotionally challenged. I've grieved at the loss of people I've
known. I remind myself daily that one day there will be an
end, and we'll be able to look back on it with wonder.
Certainly, we will all have a new perspective and deeper
understanding of human behavior and sexuality.

The happy ending, however, will only arrive if all of us
realize that this is a universal women's problem and we
can be part of the solution.

We are compassionate. We are the nurturers, the com-
municators, the teachers and the caregivers. We will
make a difference, whether it's in the boardroom or the
bedroom.

APPENDIX 1

GLOSSARY

Anatomy

Anus — The opening between the buttocks, from which the bowel movement is released.

Cervix — The lower end of the uterus, which juts into the vagina.

Clitoris — Mound of sensitive tissue at the mouth of the labia, which becomes bigger, erect or bloodfilled during sexual excitement.

Genitalia (or genitals) — The external sex organs: the penis in males; vulva, labia and clitoris in females.

Labia — Folds of skin and mucus membrane covering the vagina and urethral opening.

Penis (cock, prick, dick or shaft) — Male's external sex organ.

Placenta — Vascular organ uniting the fetus to the maternal uterus and admitting the exchange of food and waste products between mother and fetus.

Urethra — Short, straight tube carrying urine from the bladder out of the body.

Vagina (cunt, "down there") — Passageway in a woman leading from the vulva to the uterus.

Vaginal secretions — Any substance composed of blood or body cells which travel through the vagina.

Vulva — The external genitalia or sex organs of a woman, including the labia, clitoris and opening of the vagina.

Sex

Anal intercourse (buggery, sodomy, rectal sex or ass fucking) — A male inserts his penis into another person's anus.

Anilingus (rimming) — Person uses mouth or tongue to stimulate another person's anus.

Bisexual — A male or female who has sex with both males and females.

Casual contact — Contacts such as hugging, shaking hands or merely sitting on the same bus with other people.

Casual transmission — Some diseases such as a cold or the flu, are transmitted through casual or airborne contact. However, AIDS is not transmitted through casual contact.

Condoms/female — Thin, rubber bag inserted into the vagina to collect male secretions during intercourse.

Condoms/male (sheath, rubber, French letter) — Thin rubber bag worn over a man's penis to collect secretion, and thus reduce the risk of pregnancy or sexually transmitted diseases.

Cunnilingus (oral sex, licking, "go down on" or sucking) — Using the tongue to stimulate a woman's genitals.

Diaphragm — Round, latex rubber contraceptive device inserted into the vagina to cover the cervix.

Ejaculation — The discharge of semen from a man's penis.

Erection (hard-on) — The engorgement of the penis with blood.

Fellatio (cock-sucking, blow job, "giving head," "go down on," oral sex) — Using the tongue or mouth to stimulate a man's penis.

Fisting (fist fucking) — Inserting a hand into another person's vagina or rectum.

French kissing (wet kissing, deep kissing) — Kissing which involves contact and exchange of saliva.

Heterosexual — A man or a woman who is sexually attracted to a member of the opposite sex.

Homosexual/Female (lesbian, dyke) — A woman who is sexually attracted to other women.

Homosexual/male (gay, queer) — A man who is sexually attracted to other men.

Intercourse (fucking, screwing) — Sexual activity in which the penis is inserted into the vagina or rectum of another person.

Masturbation — Self-stimulation of one's genitals or other sensitive areas.

Monogamous — Having only one sex partner.

Oral sex — Sexual activity in which the male places his penis in his partner's mouth, or the woman's vaginal area is rubbed by her partner's tongue or mouth.

Safer sex — Sex which reduces the risk of infection with HIV, unwanted pregnancy and sexually transmitted diseases. There is no mucus membrane contact or bodily fluid exchange between partners.

Semen — Male body fluid containing sperm. It is ejaculated when a male has an orgasm during sexual intercourse, wet dream or masturbation.

Unprotected sex — Sexual intercourse without the use of a condom.

Vaginal intercourse (fucking, screwing, coitus, making love) — Sexual activity in which the penis is inserted into the vagina.

Water sports (golden showers) — Slang term for sexual activities that involve urine.

Wet sex — Any kind of behavior in which bodily fluids are exchanged.

Drugs/Pharmacology

AZT (Retrovir or Zidovudine), DDI or DDC — Drugs which have helped extend the lives of people with AIDS. They cannot cure the disease.

Injection drugs — Drugs which are injected into the body with a needle.

Intravenous drugs — Drugs injected into the blood veins with a needle.

Lubricant — A preparation, such as KY jelly, which lessens the friction during sexual intercourse.

Nonoxynol-9 — A spermicide which is thought to deactivate the AIDS virus.

Spermicide — A contraceptive which kills sperm.

Testing

Anonymous — Without any identification which would let others know your true name.

Antibodies — Or antibody, a specific protein produced by the immune system to fight a specific infection.

Confidential — Information kept private.

ELISA — The first screening test used to find HIV antibodies in blood.

False negative HIV test — Someone infected with the AIDS virus may have a false negative result because insufficient time has passed for the body to produce enough antibodies to the virus, hence the test for HIV is negative.

False positive HIV test — A positive result from an HIV blood test, when in fact the person does not have the virus.

HIV antibody positive — A blood test result showing that a person has been infected with HIV at some time and has developed antibodies to the virus.

Seropositive — A person has antibodies to HIV.

Western Blot — A test to detect HIV antibodies in blood. It is used to confirm the ELISA test result.

Window period — The length of time between when a person is infected with HIV and when that person produces antibodies to HIV. The AIDS test screens for antibodies which take some time to develop. This means a person can be infected, yet still test negative during the window period.

General

Abstinence — Refraining from something, for example, sexual intercourse and illicit drugs.

AIDS — Acquired Immune Deficiency Syndrome, a disease which weakens the immune system's ability to fight off infections.

ARC — AIDS Related Complex, a condition caused by HIV. People with ARC have certain physical symptoms of illness, but do not have the specific infections necessary for a diagnosis of AIDS. That is, they do not have opportunistic infections or cancer. This term is no longer used by the medical profession.

Asymptomatic — Someone who is infected with HIV, but is not showing any signs or symptoms of illness.

CDC — Centers for Disease Control, a federal agency that studies, monitors and provides information on the nation's health and safety.

Contraceptive — An agent used to prevent pregnancy.

Dementia — Loss of mental capacity resulting from the progressive destruction of brain cells.

Epidemic — Outbreak of a contagious disease, attacking many people at the same time.

Epidemiology — The study of epidemics and disease transmission.

Exposure — Contact with a disease producing agents such as HIV.

FDA — Food and Drug Administration, a department of the U.S. Health and Human Services, which monitors and approves all new drugs and food products.

Hemophilia — Rare hereditary disease found predominantly in men in which the blood does not clot normally.

Hepatitis — Inflammation of the liver.

Immune system — The body's defense mechanism against infection and disease.

Kaposi's Sarcoma — Rare form of cancer showing up as pink, purple or brown spots on the skin. This cancer is common among people with AIDS.

Lymph nodes — Structures in the body whose function is to filter impurities, viruses and bacteria from the body.

Opportunistic infections — Infections caused by organisms, which people with healthy immune systems are easily able to fight off. However, they take the opportunity to infect and cause serious illnesses in people with a deficiency in their immune system.

PWA — A person with AIDS.

T-Cells — Also know as T-helper cells or CD-4 cells, they are a type of white blood cell that protect the body against forcing organisms.

Transmission — The passing of infection or disease from one person to another.

Vaccine — A substance which causes immunity or protection from a disease.

VD — Venereal diseases, diseases which are transmitted through sexual intercourse.

Virus — A very small organism, which can only be seen with a microscope. Viruses are responsible for many diseases, including the common cold and flu.

White blood cells — These are certain cells in the blood which fight against infection.

"Works" — A term used by drug users to refer to the needles, syringes and equipment used to mix and prepare drugs for illegal intravenous use.

WHO — World Health Organization, an organization that monitors worldwide health.

APPENDIX 2

$\mathcal{H}$IV/AIDS Resource Directory

The following organizations offer information concerning HIV disease or other sexually transmitted diseases. In addition, you might check with your local health department, crisis hotlines, or HIV/AIDS centers. If you have trouble finding a service, call the National AIDS Hotline which can provide you with information on a wide variety of services available in your area.

National AIDS Hotline
1-800-342-2437 (English)
1-800-344-7432 (Spanish)
1-800-243-7889 (Hearing Impaired)

Centers for Disease Control AIDS Clearinghouse
1-800-458-5231

AIDS Hotline for Teens
1-800-234-TEEN

National STD Hotline
1-800-227-8922

National Herpes Hotline
1-919-361-8488

American Red Cross AIDS Education Office
1-202-737-8300

AIDS Clinical Trials Information Service
1-800-243-7012
AIDS Treatment News
1-415-255-0588
National Association of People with AIDS
1-202-429-2856
The Positive Woman
1-202-898-0372

Support Groups

Sex and Love Addicts Anonymous (SLAA)
The Augustine Fellowship
P.O. Box 88
New Town Branch
Boston, MA 02258
(617) 332-1845

Sex Addicts Anonymous (SAA)
Adult Children of Sex Addicts Anonymous (ACSA)
P.O. Box 3038
Minneapolis, MN 55403
1-612-339-0217

Sexaholics Anonymous (SA)
P.O. Box 300
Simi Valley, CA 93062
1-818-704-9854

S-Anon (for families of sex addicts)
P.O. Box 5117
Sherman Oaks, CA 91413
1-818-990-6910

Co-Dependents Anonymous (CODA)
P.O. Box 33577
Phoenix, AZ 85067-3577
(602) 277-7991

*B*IBLIOGRAPHY

Scientific Journals And Reference Sources

Allen, M., and Marte, C. "HIV Infection in Women: Presentations and Protocols." *Hospital Practice* (March 1992); 155-162.

Anderson, J. "HIV in Women: Factors that Increase Their Risk." *Medical Aspects of Human Sexuality* (May 1991); 20-28.

Burke, D., and Brundage, J. "Human Immunodeficiency Virus Infections in Teenagers." *Journal of the American Medical Association* (April 1990); 2074-2077.

Chamberland, M. "HIV Transmission from Health Care Worker to Patient: What Is the Risk?" *Annals of Internal Medicine* (May 1992); 871-872.

Chamberland M.; Conley, L.; et al. "Health Care Workers with AIDS." *Journal of the American Medical Association* (December 1991); 3459-3462.

Chu, S.; Buehler, J.; et al. "Epidemiology of Reported Cases of AIDS in Lesbians, United States." *American Journal of Public Health* (November 1990); 1380-1381.

Chu, S.; Buehler, J.; et al. "Impact of the Human Immunodeficiency Virus Epidemic on Mortality of Women in

Reproductive Age, United States." *Journal of the American Medical Association* (July 1990); 225-229.

Dinsmoor, M. "HIV Infection and Pregnancy." *Medical Clinics of North America* (May 1989); 701-711.

Fischl, M. and Dickinson, G. "Evaluation of Heterosexual Partners, Children, and Household Contacts of Adults with AIDS." *Journal of the American Medical Association* (February 1987); 640-644.

Goodgame, R. "AIDS in Uganda — Clinical and Social Features." *New England Journal of Medicine* (August 1990); 383-388.

Jaffee, L.; Seehaus, M. et al. "Anal Intercourse and Knowledge of Acquired Immunodeficiency among Minority-Group Female Adolescents." *Journal of Pediatrics* (June 1988); 1005-1007.

Lenes, B. and Hamilton, J. "HIV Infection and the Blood Supply." *Miami Medicine* (December 1991); 17-19.

Minkoff, H. and Dehovitz, J. "Care of Women Infected with the Human Immunodeficiency Virus." *Journal of the American Medical Association* (October 1991); 2253-2257.

Novello, A. Letter from the Surgeon General, United States Public Health Service: "Women and HIV Infection." *Journal of the American Medical Association* (April 1991); 1805.

Novello, A. and Soto-Torres, L. "Women and Hidden Epidemics: HIV/AIDS and Domestic Violence." *The Female Patient* (January 1992); 17-31.

O'Brien, T. and George, R. "Human Immunodeficiency Virus Type 2 in the United States." *Journal of the American Medical Association* (May 1992); 2775-2779.

Smeltzer, S. and Whipple, B. "Women and HIV Infection." *Image: Journal of Nursing Scholarship* (Winter 1991); 249-256.

Spence, M. and Reboli, A. "Human Immunodeficiency Virus Infection in Women." *Annals of Internal Medicine* (November 1991); 827-829.

St. Louis, M.; Conway, G.; et al. "Human Immunodeficiency Infection in Disadvantaged Adolescents." *Journal of the American Medical Association* (November 1991); 2387-2391.

Extended Reading List

Adams, K.M. *Silently Seduced.* Deerfield Beach, FL: Health Communications, 1991.

DeCotiis, S. *A Woman's Guide to Sexual Health.* New York: Pocket Books, 1989.

Hein, K. and Digeronimo, T. *AIDS: Trading Fears for Facts.* Yonkers, NY: Consumers Union of United States, Inc., 1989.

Hite, S. *The Hite Report on Male Sexuality.* New York: Ballantine Books, 1982.

Hite, S. *Women and Love.* New York: St. Martin's Press, 1989.

Kaplan, H. *The Real Truth About Women and AIDS.* New York: Simon & Schuster, 1987.

Miller, N. and Rockwell, R. *AIDS in Africa: The Social and Policy Impact.* Lewiston, NY: The Edwin Mellen Press, 1989.

Money, J. *How to Persuade Your Lover to Use a Condom . . . And Why You Should.* San Francisco: New York Publishing, 1987.

Norwood, C. *Advice for Life.* New York: Pantheon Books, 1987.

Panos Institute. *Triple Jeopardy: Women and AIDS.* Washington, D.C.: Panos Publications, Ltd., 1990.

Petrow, S. *Ending the HIV Epidemic*. Santa Cruz, Calif.: Network Publications, 1990.

Richardson, D. *Women and the AIDS Crisis*. Winchester, Mass.: Unwin Hyman, Ltd., 1989.

Vaughan, P. *The Monogamy Myth*. New York: Newmarket Press, 1989.